Mometrix
TEST PREPARATION

Secrets of the

ARDMS®

Obstetrics and Gynecology Exam Study Guide

DEAR FUTURE EXAM SUCCESS STORY

First of all, **THANK YOU** for purchasing Mometrix study materials!

Second, congratulations! You are one of the few determined test-takers who are committed to doing whatever it takes to excel on your exam. **You have come to the right place.** We developed these study materials with one goal in mind: to deliver you the information you need in a format that's concise and easy to use.

In addition to optimizing your guide for the content of the test, we've outlined our recommended steps for breaking down the preparation process into small, attainable goals so you can make sure you stay on track.

We've also analyzed the entire test-taking process, identifying the most common pitfalls and showing how you can overcome them and be ready for any curveball the test throws you.

Standardized testing is one of the biggest obstacles on your road to success, which only increases the importance of doing well in the high-pressure, high-stakes environment of test day. Your results on this test could have a significant impact on your future, and this guide provides the information and practical advice to help you achieve your full potential on test day.

Your success is our success

We would love to hear from you! If you would like to share the story of your exam success or if you have any questions or comments in regard to our products, please contact us at **800-673-8175** or **support@mometrix.com**.

Thanks again for your business and we wish you continued success!

Sincerely,
The Mometrix Test Preparation Team

Need more help? Check out our flashcards at:
http://MometrixFlashcards.com/ARDMS

Written and edited by the Mometrix Exam Secrets Test Prep Team
Printed in the United States of America

TABLE OF CONTENTS

INTRODUCTION 1

SECRET KEY #1 – PLAN BIG, STUDY SMALL 2

SECRET KEY #2 – MAKE YOUR STUDYING COUNT 3

SECRET KEY #3 – PRACTICE THE RIGHT WAY 4

SECRET KEY #4 – PACE YOURSELF 6

SECRET KEY #5 – HAVE A PLAN FOR GUESSING 7

TEST-TAKING STRATEGIES 10

GYNECOLOGY 15
- NORMAL ANATOMY AND PHYSIOLOGY 15
- ABNORMAL PHYSIOLOGY AND PERFUSION 20

OBSTETRICS - FIRST TRIMESTER 32
- NORMAL ANATOMY AND PHYSIOLOGY 32
- ABNORMALITIES AND COMPLICATIONS 38

OBSTETRICS - SECOND/THIRD TRIMESTER 46
- NORMAL ANATOMY AND PHYSIOLOGY 46
- FETAL ABNORMALITIES 56
- PLACENTAL AND UMBILICAL ABNORMALITIES 78
- CERVIX AND MATERNAL PATHOLOGY 83

PROTOCOLS AND PROCEDURES 87
- CLINICAL STANDARDS AND GUIDELINES 87
- MEASUREMENT TECHNIQUES 89
- SONOGRAPHER ROLE IN PROCEDURES 95

PHYSICS AND INSTRUMENTATION 100
- HEMODYNAMICS 100
- IMAGING INSTRUMENTS 102

ARDMS PRACTICE TEST 107

ANSWER KEY AND EXPLANATIONS 115

HOW TO OVERCOME TEST ANXIETY 123

ONLINE RESOURCES 130

Introduction

Thank you for purchasing this resource! You have made the choice to prepare yourself for a test that could have a huge impact on your future, and this guide is designed to help you be fully ready for test day. Obviously, it's important to have a solid understanding of the test material, but you also need to be prepared for the unique environment and stressors of the test, so that you can perform to the best of your abilities.

For this purpose, the first section that appears in this guide is the **Secret Keys**. We've devoted countless hours to meticulously researching what works and what doesn't, and we've boiled down our findings to the five most impactful steps you can take to improve your performance on the test. We start at the beginning with study planning and move through the preparation process, all the way to the testing strategies that will help you get the most out of what you know when you're finally sitting in front of the test.

We recommend that you start preparing for your test as far in advance as possible. However, if you've bought this guide as a last-minute study resource and only have a few days before your test, we recommend that you skip over the first two Secret Keys since they address a long-term study plan.

If you struggle with **test anxiety**, we strongly encourage you to check out our recommendations for how you can overcome it. Test anxiety is a formidable foe, but it can be beaten, and we want to make sure you have the tools you need to defeat it.

Secret Key #1 – Plan Big, Study Small

There's a lot riding on your performance. If you want to ace this test, you're going to need to keep your skills sharp and the material fresh in your mind. You need a plan that lets you review everything you need to know while still fitting in your schedule. We'll break this strategy down into three categories.

Information Organization

Start with the information you already have: the official test outline. From this, you can make a complete list of all the concepts you need to cover before the test. Organize these concepts into groups that can be studied together, and create a list of any related vocabulary you need to learn so you can brush up on any difficult terms. You'll want to keep this vocabulary list handy once you actually start studying since you may need to add to it along the way.

Time Management

Once you have your set of study concepts, decide how to spread them out over the time you have left before the test. Break your study plan into small, clear goals so you have a manageable task for each day and know exactly what you're doing. Then just focus on one small step at a time. When you manage your time this way, you don't need to spend hours at a time studying. Studying a small block of content for a short period each day helps you retain information better and avoid stressing over how much you have left to do. You can relax knowing that you have a plan to cover everything in time. In order for this strategy to be effective though, you have to start studying early and stick to your schedule. Avoid the exhaustion and futility that comes from last-minute cramming!

Study Environment

The environment you study in has a big impact on your learning. Studying in a coffee shop, while probably more enjoyable, is not likely to be as fruitful as studying in a quiet room. It's important to keep distractions to a minimum. You're only planning to study for a short block of time, so make the most of it. Don't pause to check your phone or get up to find a snack. It's also important to **avoid multitasking**. Research has consistently shown that multitasking will make your studying dramatically less effective. Your study area should also be comfortable and well-lit so you don't have the distraction of straining your eyes or sitting on an uncomfortable chair.

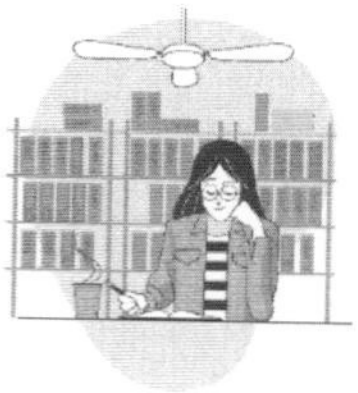

The time of day you study is also important. You want to be rested and alert. Don't wait until just before bedtime. Study when you'll be most likely to comprehend and remember. Even better, if you know what time of day your test will be, set that time aside for study. That way your brain will be used to working on that subject at that specific time and you'll have a better chance of recalling information.

Finally, it can be helpful to team up with others who are studying for the same test. Your actual studying should be done in as isolated an environment as possible, but the work of organizing the information and setting up the study plan can be divided up. In between study sessions, you can discuss with your teammates the concepts that you're all studying and quiz each other on the details. Just be sure that your teammates are as serious about the test as you are. If you find that your study time is being replaced with social time, you might need to find a new team.

Secret Key #2 – Make Your Studying Count

You're devoting a lot of time and effort to preparing for this test, so you want to be absolutely certain it will pay off. This means doing more than just reading the content and hoping you can remember it on test day. It's important to make every minute of study count. There are two main areas you can focus on to make your studying count.

Retention

It doesn't matter how much time you study if you can't remember the material. You need to make sure you are retaining the concepts. To check your retention of the information you're learning, try recalling it at later times with minimal prompting. Try carrying around flashcards and glance at one or two from time to time or ask a friend who's also studying for the test to quiz you.

To enhance your retention, look for ways to put the information into practice so that you can apply it rather than simply recalling it. If you're using the information in practical ways, it will be much easier to remember. Similarly, it helps to solidify a concept in your mind if you're not only reading it to yourself but also explaining it to someone else. Ask a friend to let you teach them about a concept you're a little shaky on (or speak aloud to an imaginary audience if necessary). As you try to summarize, define, give examples, and answer your friend's questions, you'll understand the concepts better and they will stay with you longer. Finally, step back for a big picture view and ask yourself how each piece of information fits with the whole subject. When you link the different concepts together and see them working together as a whole, it's easier to remember the individual components.

Finally, practice showing your work on any multi-step problems, even if you're just studying. Writing out each step you take to solve a problem will help solidify the process in your mind, and you'll be more likely to remember it during the test.

Modality

Modality simply refers to the means or method by which you study. Choosing a study modality that fits your own individual learning style is crucial. No two people learn best in exactly the same way, so it's important to know your strengths and use them to your advantage.

For example, if you learn best by visualization, focus on visualizing a concept in your mind and draw an image or a diagram. Try color-coding your notes, illustrating them, or creating symbols that will trigger your mind to recall a learned concept. If you learn best by hearing or discussing information, find a study partner who learns the same way or read aloud to yourself. Think about how to put the information in your own words. Imagine that you are giving a lecture on the topic and record yourself so you can listen to it later.

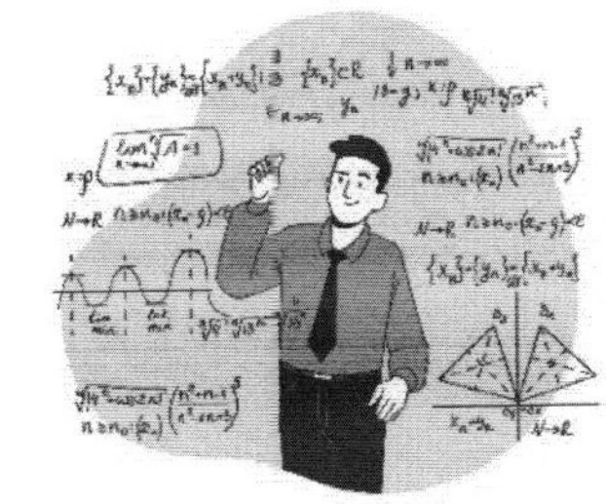

For any learning style, flashcards can be helpful. Organize the information so you can take advantage of spare moments to review. Underline key words or phrases. Use different colors for different categories. Mnemonic devices (such as creating a short list in which every item starts with the same letter) can also help with retention. Find what works best for you and use it to store the information in your mind most effectively and easily.

Secret Key #3 – Practice the Right Way

Your success on test day depends not only on how many hours you put into preparing, but also on whether you prepared the right way. It's good to check along the way to see if your studying is paying off. One of the most effective ways to do this is by taking practice tests to evaluate your progress. Practice tests are useful because they show exactly where you need to improve. Every time you take a practice test, pay special attention to these three groups of questions:

- The questions you got wrong
- The questions you had to guess on, even if you guessed right
- The questions you found difficult or slow to work through

This will show you exactly what your weak areas are, and where you need to devote more study time. Ask yourself why each of these questions gave you trouble. Was it because you didn't understand the material? Was it because you didn't remember the vocabulary? Do you need more repetitions on this type of question to build speed and confidence? Dig into those questions and figure out how you can strengthen your weak areas as you go back to review the material.

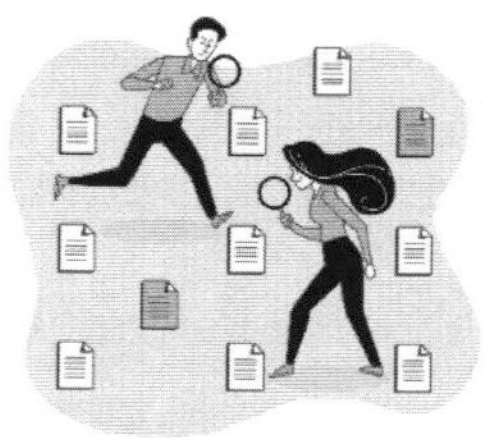

Additionally, many practice tests have a section explaining the answer choices. It can be tempting to read the explanation and think that you now have a good understanding of the concept. However, an explanation likely only covers part of the question's broader context. Even if the explanation makes perfect sense, **go back and investigate** every concept related to the question until you're positive you have a thorough understanding.

As you go along, keep in mind that the practice test is just that: practice. Memorizing these questions and answers will not be very helpful on the actual test because it is unlikely to have any of the same exact questions. If you only know the right answers to the sample questions, you won't be prepared for the real thing. **Study the concepts** until you understand them fully, and then you'll be able to answer any question that shows up on the test.

It's important to wait on the practice tests until you're ready. If you take a test on your first day of study, you may be overwhelmed by the amount of material covered and how much you need to learn. Work up to it gradually.

On test day, you'll need to be prepared for answering questions, managing your time, and using the test-taking strategies you've learned. It's a lot to balance, like a mental marathon that will have a big impact on your future. Like training for a marathon, you'll need to start slowly and work your way up. When test day arrives, you'll be ready.

Start with the strategies you've read in the first two Secret Keys—plan your course and study in the way that works best for you. If you have time, consider using multiple study resources to get different approaches to the same concepts. It can be helpful to see difficult concepts from more than one angle. Then find a good source for practice tests. Many times, the test website will suggest potential study resources or provide sample tests.

Practice Test Strategy

If you're able to find at least three practice tests, we recommend this strategy:

Untimed and Open-Book Practice

Take the first test with no time constraints and with your notes and study guide handy. Take your time and focus on applying the strategies you've learned.

Timed and Open-Book Practice

Take the second practice test open-book as well, but set a timer and practice pacing yourself to finish in time.

Timed and Closed-Book Practice

Take any other practice tests as if it were test day. Set a timer and put away your study materials. Sit at a table or desk in a quiet room, imagine yourself at the testing center, and answer questions as quickly and accurately as possible.

Keep repeating timed and closed-book tests on a regular basis until you run out of practice tests or it's time for the actual test. Your mind will be ready for the schedule and stress of test day, and you'll be able to focus on recalling the material you've learned.

Secret Key #4 – Pace Yourself

Once you're fully prepared for the material on the test, your biggest challenge on test day will be managing your time. Just knowing that the clock is ticking can make you panic even if you have plenty of time left. Work on pacing yourself so you can build confidence against the time constraints of the exam. Pacing is a difficult skill to master, especially in a high-pressure environment, so **practice is vital**.

Set time expectations for your pace based on how much time is available. For example, if a section has 60 questions and the time limit is 30 minutes, you know you have to average 30 seconds or less per question in order to answer them all. Although 30 seconds is the hard limit, set 25 seconds per question as your goal, so you reserve extra time to spend on harder questions. When you budget extra time for the harder questions, you no longer have any reason to stress when those questions take longer to answer.

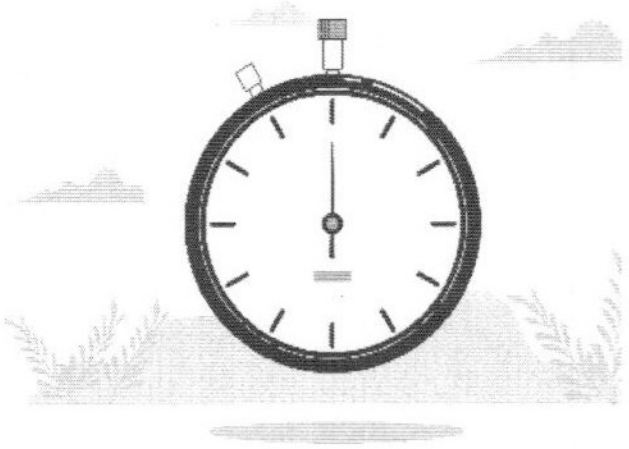

Don't let this time expectation distract you from working through the test at a calm, steady pace, but keep it in mind so you don't spend too much time on any one question. Recognize that taking extra time on one question you don't understand may keep you from answering two that you do understand later in the test. If your time limit for a question is up and you're still not sure of the answer, mark it and move on, and come back to it later if the time and the test format allow. If the testing format doesn't allow you to return to earlier questions, just make an educated guess; then put it out of your mind and move on.

On the easier questions, be careful not to rush. It may seem wise to hurry through them so you have more time for the challenging ones, but it's not worth missing one if you know the concept and just didn't take the time to read the question fully. Work efficiently but make sure you understand the question and have looked at all of the answer choices, since more than one may seem right at first.

Even if you're paying attention to the time, you may find yourself a little behind at some point. You should speed up to get back on track, but do so wisely. Don't panic; just take a few seconds less on each question until you're caught up. Don't guess without thinking, but do look through the answer choices and eliminate any you know are wrong. If you can get down to two choices, it is often worthwhile to guess from those. Once you've chosen an answer, move on and don't dwell on any that you skipped or had to hurry through. If a question was taking too long, chances are it was one of the harder ones, so you weren't as likely to get it right anyway.

On the other hand, if you find yourself getting ahead of schedule, it may be beneficial to slow down a little. The more quickly you work, the more likely you are to make a careless mistake that will affect your score. You've budgeted time for each question, so don't be afraid to spend that time. Practice an efficient but careful pace to get the most out of the time you have.

Secret Key #5 – Have a Plan for Guessing

When you're taking the test, you may find yourself stuck on a question. Some of the answer choices seem better than others, but you don't see the one answer choice that is obviously correct. What do you do?

The scenario described above is very common, yet most test takers have not effectively prepared for it. Developing and practicing a plan for guessing may be one of the single most effective uses of your time as you get ready for the exam.

In developing your plan for guessing, there are three questions to address:

- When should you start the guessing process?
- How should you narrow down the choices?
- Which answer should you choose?

When to Start the Guessing Process

Unless your plan for guessing is to select C every time (which, despite its merits, is not what we recommend), you need to leave yourself enough time to apply your answer elimination strategies. Since you have a limited amount of time for each question, that means that if you're going to give yourself the best shot at guessing correctly, you have to decide quickly whether or not you will guess.

Of course, the best-case scenario is that you don't have to guess at all, so first, see if you can answer the question based on your knowledge of the subject and basic reasoning skills. Focus on the key words in the question and try to jog your memory of related topics. Give yourself a chance to bring the knowledge to mind, but once you realize that you don't have (or you can't access) the knowledge you need to answer the question, it's time to start the guessing process.

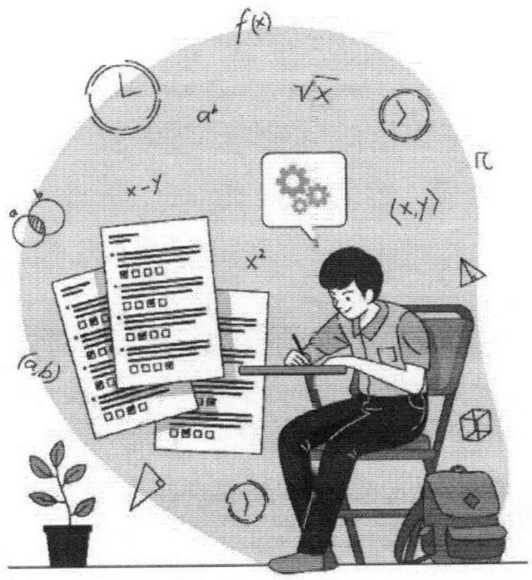

It's almost always better to start the guessing process too early than too late. It only takes a few seconds to remember something and answer the question from knowledge. Carefully eliminating wrong answer choices takes longer. Plus, going through the process of eliminating answer choices can actually help jog your memory.

Summary: Start the guessing process as soon as you decide that you can't answer the question based on your knowledge.

How to Narrow Down the Choices

The next chapter in this book (**Test-Taking Strategies**) includes a wide range of strategies for how to approach questions and how to look for answer choices to eliminate. You will definitely want to read those carefully, practice them, and figure out which ones work best for you. Here though, we're going to address a mindset rather than a particular strategy.

Your odds of guessing an answer correctly depend on how many options you are choosing from.

Number of options left	5	4	3	2	1
Odds of guessing correctly	20%	25%	33%	50%	100%

You can see from this chart just how valuable it is to be able to eliminate incorrect answers and make an educated guess, but there are two things that many test takers do that cause them to miss out on the benefits of guessing:

- Accidentally eliminating the correct answer
- Selecting an answer based on an impression

We'll look at the first one here, and the second one in the next section.

To avoid accidentally eliminating the correct answer, we recommend a thought exercise called **the $5 challenge**. In this challenge, you only eliminate an answer choice from contention if you are willing to bet $5 on it being wrong. Why $5? Five dollars is a small but not insignificant amount of money. It's an amount you could afford to lose but wouldn't want to throw away. And while losing $5 once might not hurt too much, doing it twenty times will set you back $100. In the same way, each small decision you make—eliminating a choice here, guessing on a question there—won't by itself impact your score very much, but when you put them all together, they can make a big difference. By holding each answer choice elimination decision to a higher standard, you can reduce the risk of accidentally eliminating the correct answer.

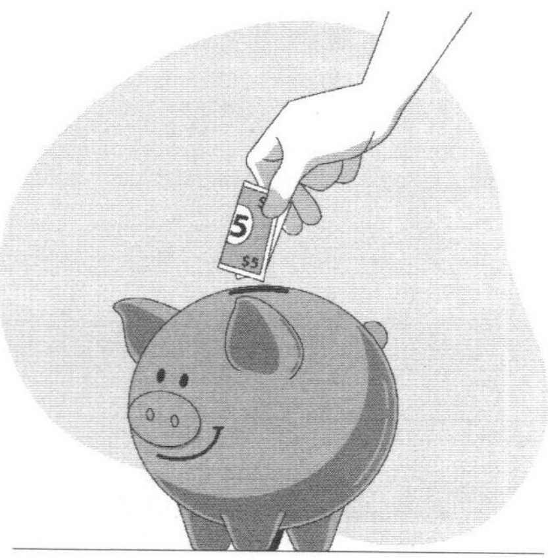

The $5 challenge can also be applied in a positive sense: If you are willing to bet $5 that an answer choice *is* correct, go ahead and mark it as correct.

Summary: Only eliminate an answer choice if you are willing to bet $5 that it is wrong.

Which Answer to Choose

You're taking the test. You've run into a hard question and decided you'll have to guess. You've eliminated all the answer choices you're willing to bet $5 on. Now you have to pick an answer. Why do we even need to talk about this? Why can't you just pick whichever one you feel like when the time comes?

The answer to these questions is that if you don't come into the test with a plan, you'll rely on your impression to select an answer choice, and if you do that, you risk falling into a trap. The test writers know that everyone who takes their test will be guessing on some of the questions, so they intentionally write wrong answer choices to seem plausible. You still have to pick an answer though, and if the wrong answer choices are designed to look right, how can you ever be sure that you're not falling for their trap? The best solution we've found to this dilemma is to take the decision out of your hands entirely. Here is the process we recommend:

Once you've eliminated any choices that you are confident (willing to bet $5) are wrong, select the first remaining choice as your answer.

Whether you choose to select the first remaining choice, the second, or the last, the important thing is that you use some preselected standard. Using this approach guarantees that you will not be enticed into selecting an answer choice that looks right, because you are not basing your decision on how the answer choices look.

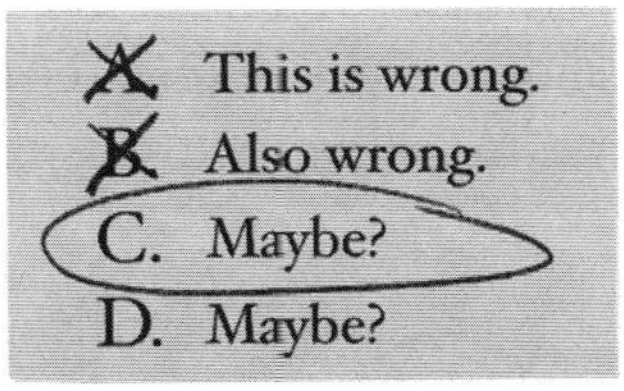

This is not meant to make you question your knowledge. Instead, it is to help you recognize the difference between your knowledge and your impressions. There's a huge difference between thinking an answer is right because of what you know, and thinking an answer is right because it looks or sounds like it should be right.

Summary: To ensure that your selection is appropriately random, make a predetermined selection from among all answer choices you have not eliminated.

Test-Taking Strategies

This section contains a list of test-taking strategies that you may find helpful as you work through the test. By taking what you know and applying logical thought, you can maximize your chances of answering any question correctly!

It is very important to realize that every question is different and every person is different: no single strategy will work on every question, and no single strategy will work for every person. That's why we've included all of them here, so you can try them out and determine which ones work best for different types of questions and which ones work best for you.

Question Strategies

✓ Read Carefully

Read the question and the answer choices carefully. Don't miss the question because you misread the terms. You have plenty of time to read each question thoroughly and make sure you understand what is being asked. Yet a happy medium must be attained, so don't waste too much time. You must read carefully and efficiently.

✓ Contextual Clues

Look for contextual clues. If the question includes a word you are not familiar with, look at the immediate context for some indication of what the word might mean. Contextual clues can often give you all the information you need to decipher the meaning of an unfamiliar word. Even if you can't determine the meaning, you may be able to narrow down the possibilities enough to make a solid guess at the answer to the question.

✓ Prefixes

If you're having trouble with a word in the question or answer choices, try dissecting it. Take advantage of every clue that the word might include. Prefixes can be a huge help. Usually, they allow you to determine a basic meaning. *Pre-* means before, *post-* means after, *pro-* is positive, *de-* is negative. From prefixes, you can get an idea of the general meaning of the word and try to put it into context.

✓ Hedge Words

Watch out for critical hedge words, such as *likely, may, can, often, almost, mostly, usually, generally, rarely,* and *sometimes.* Question writers insert these hedge phrases to cover every possibility. Often an answer choice will be wrong simply because it leaves no room for exception. Be on guard for answer choices that have definitive words such as *exactly* and *always.*

✓ Switchback Words

Stay alert for *switchbacks.* These are the words and phrases frequently used to alert you to shifts in thought. The most common switchback words are *but, although,* and *however.* Others include *nevertheless, on the other hand, even though, while, in spite of, despite,* and *regardless of.* Switchback words are important to catch because they can change the direction of the question or an answer choice.

✓ FACE VALUE

When in doubt, use common sense. Accept the situation in the problem at face value. Don't read too much into it. These problems will not require you to make wild assumptions. If you have to go beyond creativity and warp time or space in order to have an answer choice fit the question, then you should move on and consider the other answer choices. These are normal problems rooted in reality. The applicable relationship or explanation may not be readily apparent, but it is there for you to figure out. Use your common sense to interpret anything that isn't clear.

Answer Choice Strategies

✓ ANSWER SELECTION

The most thorough way to pick an answer choice is to identify and eliminate wrong answers until only one is left, then confirm it is the correct answer. Sometimes an answer choice may immediately seem right, but be careful. The test writers will usually put more than one reasonable answer choice on each question, so take a second to read all of them and make sure that the other choices are not equally obvious. As long as you have time left, it is better to read every answer choice than to pick the first one that looks right without checking the others.

✓ ANSWER CHOICE FAMILIES

An answer choice family consists of two (in rare cases, three) answer choices that are very similar in construction and cannot all be true at the same time. If you see two answer choices that are direct opposites or parallels, one of them is usually the correct answer. For instance, if one answer choice says that quantity *x* increases and another either says that quantity *x* decreases (opposite) or says that quantity *y* increases (parallel), then those answer choices would fall into the same family. An answer choice that doesn't match the construction of the answer choice family is more likely to be incorrect. Most questions will not have answer choice families, but when they do appear, you should be prepared to recognize them.

✓ ELIMINATE ANSWERS

Eliminate answer choices as soon as you realize they are wrong, but make sure you consider all possibilities. If you are eliminating answer choices and realize that the last one you are left with is also wrong, don't panic. Start over and consider each choice again. There may be something you missed the first time that you will realize on the second pass.

✓ AVOID FACT TRAPS

Don't be distracted by an answer choice that is factually true but doesn't answer the question. You are looking for the choice that answers the question. Stay focused on what the question is asking for so you don't accidentally pick an answer that is true but incorrect. Always go back to the question and make sure the answer choice you've selected actually answers the question and is not merely a true statement.

✓ EXTREME STATEMENTS

In general, you should avoid answers that put forth extreme actions as standard practice or proclaim controversial ideas as established fact. An answer choice that states the "process should be used in certain situations, if..." is much more likely to be correct than one that states the "process should be discontinued completely." The first is a calm rational statement and doesn't even make a definitive, uncompromising stance, using a hedge word *if* to provide wiggle room, whereas the second choice is far more extreme.

⊘ BENCHMARK

As you read through the answer choices and you come across one that seems to answer the question well, mentally select that answer choice. This is not your final answer, but it's the one that will help you evaluate the other answer choices. The one that you selected is your benchmark or standard for judging each of the other answer choices. Every other answer choice must be compared to your benchmark. That choice is correct until proven otherwise by another answer choice beating it. If you find a better answer, then that one becomes your new benchmark. Once you've decided that no other choice answers the question as well as your benchmark, you have your final answer.

⊘ PREDICT THE ANSWER

Before you even start looking at the answer choices, it is often best to try to predict the answer. When you come up with the answer on your own, it is easier to avoid distractions and traps because you will know exactly what to look for. The right answer choice is unlikely to be word-for-word what you came up with, but it should be a close match. Even if you are confident that you have the right answer, you should still take the time to read each option before moving on.

General Strategies

⊘ TOUGH QUESTIONS

If you are stumped on a problem or it appears too hard or too difficult, don't waste time. Move on! Remember though, if you can quickly check for obviously incorrect answer choices, your chances of guessing correctly are greatly improved. Before you completely give up, at least try to knock out a couple of possible answers. Eliminate what you can and then guess at the remaining answer choices before moving on.

⊘ CHECK YOUR WORK

Since you will probably not know every term listed and the answer to every question, it is important that you get credit for the ones that you do know. Don't miss any questions through careless mistakes. If at all possible, try to take a second to look back over your answer selection and make sure you've selected the correct answer choice and haven't made a costly careless mistake (such as marking an answer choice that you didn't mean to mark). This quick double check should more than pay for itself in caught mistakes for the time it costs.

⊘ PACE YOURSELF

It's easy to be overwhelmed when you're looking at a page full of questions; your mind is confused and full of random thoughts, and the clock is ticking down faster than you would like. Calm down and maintain the pace that you have set for yourself. Especially as you get down to the last few minutes of the test, don't let the small numbers on the clock make you panic. As long as you are on track by monitoring your pace, you are guaranteed to have time for each question.

⊘ DON'T RUSH

It is very easy to make errors when you are in a hurry. Maintaining a fast pace in answering questions is pointless if it makes you miss questions that you would have gotten right otherwise. Test writers like to include distracting information and wrong answers that seem right. Taking a little extra time to avoid careless mistakes can make all the difference in your test score. Find a pace that allows you to be confident in the answers that you select.

✓ KEEP MOVING

Panicking will not help you pass the test, so do your best to stay calm and keep moving. Taking deep breaths and going through the answer elimination steps you practiced can help to break through a stress barrier and keep your pace.

Final Notes

The combination of a solid foundation of content knowledge and the confidence that comes from practicing your plan for applying that knowledge is the key to maximizing your performance on test day. As your foundation of content knowledge is built up and strengthened, you'll find that the strategies included in this chapter become more and more effective in helping you quickly sift through the distractions and traps of the test to isolate the correct answer.

Now that you're preparing to move forward into the test content chapters of this book, be sure to keep your goal in mind. As you read, think about how you will be able to apply this information on the test. If you've already seen sample questions for the test and you have an idea of the question format and style, try to come up with questions of your own that you can answer based on what you're reading. This will give you valuable practice applying your knowledge in the same ways you can expect to on test day.

Good luck and good studying!

Gynecology

Normal Anatomy and Physiology

Urinary Bladder and Colon

Initially, the urinary bladder is best evaluated with the transabdominal technique due to its anterior anatomical location to the uterus. Urinary bladder retention and mass may be evaluated as well as abnormalities associated with the ureters. Ureters should be sonographically evaluated for stones, ureteroceles and dilation. Endovaginal sonography technique may be useful if these structures are not adequately described with transabdominal technique. The sigmoid colon is best visualized with endovaginal sonographic technique due to it posterior location to the uterus. On sonography, the sigmoid colon usually appears echogenic with shadowing. Adequate assessment of this area may be dependent on the presence or absence of bowel.

Uterine Development

The uterus develops from Müllerian ducts that form the fallopian tubes. In normal cases, the fused ducts form the fallopian tubes and then the body of the uterus. Abnormal fusion of ducts leads to a variety of uterine malformations. From birth to about two years of age, the uterus slightly decreases in size. From the age of two to ten, the uterus takes on the size and shape of a pear. It remains a similar overall length measurement (3 cm) during this time, but the distribution changes. The uterus of a child has an equal ratio of uterine body length to cervix length. The ratio of uterine body length to cervix length doubles to triples at puberty. From about 10 to 13 years of age, the total length of the uterus increases about 2 – 2.5 cm from its childhood length.

Nonparous Uterus Sonographic Exam

In the nonparous female, a pelvic and transvaginal ultrasound may be performed. The pelvic portion gives an "overview" of pelvic structure, while the transvaginal approach allows for more detailed documentation of measurement and texture of structures. The size (in all major planes), angle, ratio, patency and positioning of associated structures of the uterus are documented. Major uterine anatomy includes the cervix, corpus (uterine body), cornu (where fallopian tubes enter uterus), and the fundus (above the cornu). Description of the thickness of the layers of the uterine wall should be included with emphasis on the innermost layer (endometrium) and the myometrium. The endometrium thickness can be dependent on the menstrual cycle, so LMP (last menstrual period) should be documented. Description of vasculature and of structures and spaces immediately outside the uterus are often documented (cul-de-sac of Douglas and vesicouterine pouch), especially if they contain fluid or are surrounded by adhesions.

Sonographic Appearance of Uterus

The sonographic appearance of the uterus should be uniform in composition and structure. Although the uterus itself is hypoechoic, the actual endometrium is echogenic. The amount of echogenicity is dependent on stage of menstrual cycle. Sonographic shadows are common on the edges of the uterus due to the network of muscular and ligamentous attachment surrounding the uterus. The broad ligament, of the uterus, contains the primary vasculature network. Sonographically, these are best visualized near the cervix and inferior most portion of the uterus. Sonographically, the fallopian tubes are difficult to visualize unless they contain pathologic findings.

Intrauterine Device Considerations

An IUD (intrauterine device) may be inserted into the endometrium for contraception. It is a highly effective method of contraception; however, it incurs some increased risk for certain disorders. It may increase the likelihood of ectopic pregnancy and pelvic inflammatory disease. Sonography may be used to assess position of IUD after placement, or if symptoms arise shortly after its insertion. It also may be an incidental finding in a sonography, although thorough patient history should decrease this likelihood. The IUD is very echogenic on ultrasound examination, thus usually easily seen. However, if clotting or products of conception remain in the endometrium, sonographic imaging may be difficult. It appears as a line, and sometimes a group of parallel lines secondary to shadows and echoes from the surface of the IUD. If the IUD is not centrally located, increased concern for implantation into the myometrium should exist.

The Endometrium

The endometrium is a key feature of the monthly menstrual cycle and reproduction. The endometrium is the inner most mucosal layer of the fallopian tubes, uterus and vagina. In addition to its importance in the cycles, the endometrium is simply important for maintaining patency of the structures with which it lines. The thickness of the endometrium varies greatly depending on the stage of menstrual or reproductive cycle, so it is important to note this stage with sonographic evaluations. During the menstrual cycle, the endometrial lining is primarily estrogenic. If ovulation occurs, the balance shifts to that of a more progestational endometrial state. Sonographically, the entire endometrium is echogenic from post ovulation to menses. From menses to ovulation (proliferative phase), the thickened endometrium is hyperechoic at the periphery and the endometrial line being echogenic.

Appearance of Endometrium

The endometrium progressively thickens throughout the phases of the menstrual cycle. The endometrial lining can be as thin as 1 mm at the beginning of menstruation to as thick as 28 mm at the luteal phase. The most sonographic change is seen within the follicular phase. At its thinnest, the endometrium is echogenic. Later in the follicular phase the endometrial stripe becomes hypoechoic. At the latest follicular phase and during ovulation, the endometrium actually appears to have three layers. These layers are echogenic on either end, with the middle layer being hypoechoic. During the luteal or secretory phase, when the endometrium is at its thickest, the appearance is strictly echogenic.

Assessment of Cervix During Pelvic Ultrasound

The cervix is the lower portion of the uterus and is located just above the vagina. To visualize the cervix during a transabdominal pelvic ultrasound, the patient must have a full bladder. This typically provides a good acoustic window, but care must be taken if the length of the cervix is to be measured. A completely full bladder may improve visualization of the cervix while increasing the cervical length. This is especially important during the obstetrical (OB) ultrasound that is ordered to determine cervical incompetence. Cervical incompetence is demonstrated by a short cervix, so this must be considered during a transabdominal ultrasound (TAUS) approach. A transvaginal ultrasound (TVUS) or endovaginal ultrasound (EVUS) approach will require the patient to empty her bladder, and the measurement is taken between the internal and external cervical os. Yet another approach that can be used to visualize the cervix is a translabial technique, which is used if a patient is having any discomfort from the EVUS or TVUS method.

Normal Position of Ovaries

Ovarian position changes after pregnancy and is not thought to return to its pregravidic state. One ovary is found on either side of the uterus, each near the lateral wall of the pelvic cavity. The ovaries are situated inferior to the fallopian tubes and attach to the posterior side of the uterine broad ligament. Each ovary is contained within the ovarian fossa, a space created at the lateral pelvic wall. The external iliac vessels support the fossa superiorly, posteriorly by the ureter, and anteriorly by the umbilical artery. It is thought that the oval ovary is positioned in a vertical manner. The suspensory ligament of the ovary is on the superior end and contains the ovarian vessels. The ligament of the ovary, within the broad uterine ligament, attaches the inferior end of the ovary to the angle of the uterus.

Menstruating Ovaries

Usually pelvic and transvaginal ultrasound are both used to evaluate the ovaries; however, the transvaginal image often assesses the ovaries more completely. It is possible that neither ultrasound will visualize the ovary. The ovaries are generally visualized posteriorly and laterally to the broad ligament; however, several anatomical variations exist. The ovary itself is shaped like an oval or ellipse and is echogenic. The multiple follicles within the ovary are hypoechoic and should be less than 3 cm. Normal sonographic appearance of the ovary depends heavily on where the patient is in relation to her menstrual cycle. Prior to ovulation, it is not unusual for a single follicle to be greater in size than surrounding follicles, up to 2.5 cm.

Fallopian Tubes

Fallopian tubes, also called uterine tubes or salpinges, arise from the Müllerian ducts. The fallopian tubes are comprised of three main sections. The first section is the portion that connects the fallopian tubes to the lateral fundus of the uterus bilaterally. This section is the proximal-most portion defined by and narrow (near the uterus) and a straight isthmus (wider section as it moves distal to the uterus). The second section is the middle portion called the ampulla. The ampulla is the usual site of fertilization. The third section of the fallopian tubes is called the infundibulum. The infundibulum is the most distal portion of the fallopian tubes and is defined by its fimbriae at the end. The fimbriae are classically described as finger like projections. The fimbriae do not directly attach to the ovaries, but they aid in collecting the egg released by the ovary, for transport down the fallopian tubes.

The Cul-De-Sac

There is an anterior cul-de-sac and a posterior cul-de-sac, which themselves are really spaces or cavities as opposed to organs or structures. The anterior cul-de-sac is space between the pubic bone and uterus, with the bladder making up the bottom of this area. The posterior cul-de-sac is also called the pouch of Douglas. The pouch of Douglas is located posterior to the uterus. Making up the other borders of the posterior cul-de-sac are: superior portion of vagina, cervix, rectum and the uterosacral ligaments. The cul-de-sacs are frequent sites of infection and endometriosis, especially the pouch of Douglas. Although this area may be difficult to view with sonography techniques, it should always be evaluated and noted for the presence of mass or fluid. If either of these findings is present, they should be clearly defined and masses should be differentiated from bowel if possible.

Normal Adult Uterus

From puberty through the teenage years, the uterine growth (along its longest axis) is up to about 3 more centimeters. the adult uterus weighs about 15 grams. at this stage the body of the uterus measures about 8 cm by 4 cm, while the cervix measures about 3 cm. The ratio of uterine body to cervix height is approximately 3:1 at this stage. The adult uterus is positioned centrally in the pelvic region with the urinary bladder anterior to it and rectum posterior to it. The broad ligaments attach to either side of the uterus laterally. There are several other smaller ligamentous networks that keep the uterus in its anatomical position.

Postmenopausal Uterus

In the postmenopausal woman that is not on hormone replacement therapy, the sonographic appearance of her uterus will be much smaller than that of a premenopausal woman. The first thing to decrease in size is the muscular portion of the body of the uterus. By about five years, post-menopause, the ratio of length of uterine body to cervix is 1:1. In addition to uterine muscular shrinkage, the endometrium thins to less than 8 mm. The postmenopausal woman on hormone replacement therapy will maintain the sonographic uterine dimensions and appearance of an adult, premenopausal female.

Postmenopausal Ovaries

Postmenopause finds the ovaries no longer ovulating and no longer the primary source of estrogen and progesterone production, as this tapers significantly during menopause and eventually ceases. The primary estrogen production then shifts to the fat cells of the body, but the rate of production is less than half of that of what the ovaries had produced. As a result of decreased hormonal production, the ovary shrinks. Typically, a postmenopausal ovary should not be larger than 2 cm along its long axis. Due to decreasing function and size, postmenopausal ovaries may be hard to detect with ultrasound. As a result of their decreasing function, they are also without many surrounding cysts that are often found around even a "normal" premenopause ovary. Hormone replacement therapy does not affect the sonographic appearance of postmenopausal ovaries.

Assessing Premenarchal Patients with Ultrasound

Menarche refers to a female's first menstrual period, often occurring between the ages of 11 and 14. Premenarchal refers to the time prior to the start of menstruation. Because most girls are virginal in this stage, transvaginal ultrasound (TVUS) is contraindicated, and, therefore, the transabdominal ultrasound (TAUS) technique should be used. This is performed while the patient has a full bladder to provide an optimal acoustic window. Anatomical structures that are identified during a pelvic ultrasound are the vagina, cervix, uterus, endometrium, ovaries, and bilateral adnexal regions. The anterior and posterior cul-de-sacs are also evaluated for the presence of free fluid. A quick survey of the patient's urinary bladder may also be performed. The advantage of a TAUS study over a TVUS study in this patient population is that it will allow for a wide field of view to provide a sufficient survey of the false pelvis during the postvoid portion of the exam. Any pathology that may have been shifted into the false pelvis by the distended bladder may be seen with this method.

Premenarchal patients have not yet started their menstrual periods. Physicians may find it necessary to evaluate the pelvic organs in young patients for many reasons that include ambiguous genitalia (which is often noticed at birth), pelvic pain, palpable mass, or amenorrhea. Ultrasound findings in these situations may include an ovarian cyst or tumor, ovarian torsion, or an absent uterus. It is important to realize that neonatal females that are scanned may demonstrate a uterus or ovaries that are enlarged due to the effect of hormones from their mother. Around the ages of seven or eight, the uterus and ovaries tend to increase in size. The pediatric uterus will range from about 2.5 to 4 cm in length and about 1 cm wide. The endometrium will appear as a thin echogenic line when visualized — until puberty, when the patient begins her menstrual cycle. Ultrasound users may visualize ovarian follicles at any age, but the volume of pediatric ovaries when calculated tends to be less than 1 cm^3.

Menstrual Cycle

There are four main phases of the menstrual cycle. First is menstruation, counted from the first day of vaginal bleeding and lasting up to 4 days. During menstruation, the endometrium is shed which produces bleeding. Second is the follicular or proliferative phase lasting approximately from day 5 to 13? This phase is marked by maturation of follicles in the ovary by initially releasing FSH from the pituitary, then LH and estradiol. Estrogen then initiates formation of a proliferative layer of endometrium. Third is ovulation, approximately day 14, marked by a surge of LH and FSH. A mature ovarian follicle ruptures, releasing an egg. Fourth, the luteal or secretory phase is approximately day 15-28. The luteal phase is marked by a surge of progesterone, which converts the endometrial lining from a proliferative lining to a secretory lining.

Abnormal Physiology and Perfusion

Ovulation and Fertility

Causes of Infertility

Infertility is a heterosexual couple's inability to conceive after 12 months of unprotected sexual intercourse. The possible causes of infertility are numerous and this list is not exhaustive. They can be placed into 4 broad categories: any condition causing anovulation, gynecological defects (anatomical), defective spermatogenesis, and external/lifestyle factors. Anovulation contributes the greatest number of infertility sources, including: diabetes, PCOS, thyroid disorders, anorexia, infection (PID), ovarian cysts, adrenal disorders, medications, previous cancer treatments, and uterine fibroids. Anatomical defects can further be broken into acquired (Asherman's syndrome, endometriosis, and adhesions) and congenital (sickle cell disease, Turner's syndrome, Klinefelter's, and Cushing's syndrome). Defects in spermatogenesis include: decreased or absent sperm production, sperm dysfunction, varicocele, hypogonadism, infection, hypospadias, and retrograde ejaculation. External factors include: pesticide exposure, other chemical exposure (lubricants), malnutrition, emotional stress, obesity, yo-yo dieting, drugs and alcohol, smoking, age, and other medical disorders (HIV/AIDs).

Disorders of Ovulation

Anovulation is responsible for about 30% of infertility. Signs of anovulation may be changes in menstrual flow (excessive, light, or absent), irregular basal temperatures, or change in premenstrual symptoms (presence or absence of PMS). Common causes of anovulation are: excess weight gain or loss, excess exercise, frequent travel, breast feeding, stress, thyroid disorders and polycystic ovary syndrome. Conception is dependent on the release of an egg from the ovary (ovulation), which then travels through the fallopian tube to unite with a sperm. If there is lack of cyclical egg release (anovulation), it follows that there is no chance of pregnancy. So identifying and attempting to correct the disorders that would prevent this are important. Restoration of regular ovulation may be done with lifestyle changes and medication.

The fallopian tubes can contribute, directly or indirectly, to many unsuccessful fertilizations. Infections such as pelvic inflammatory disease (PID) and appendicitis can cause significant inflammation in the area. PID places a woman at high risk for developing an ectopic pregnancy, which in itself is a contributor to infertility. Ectopic pregnancy is a result of a fertilized egg and sperm implanting themselves within the fallopian tube rather than the uterus, this most commonly happens at the ampulla. Furthermore, endometriosis and adhesions can contribute to decreased patency and function of the fallopian tubes, leading to infertility. Elective infertility involving the fallopian tubes is a common occurrence. In a tubal ligation, or female sterilization procedure, the tubes are either "tied", a section removed, a section removed and tied, or severed.

Upper Abdominal Findings

In addition to referred pain, the upper abdomen may contain clues to pelvic pathology on sonographic examination. Ovarian cancer should be considered if widespread serous fluid is imaged in the peritoneum or if a mass is imaged in the omental tissue. If liver metastases are sonographed, consider a primary cancer in the distal colon. Pelvic mass, inflammation, or pathology may affect the ureters, thus the demonstration of dilated kidney(s) on ultrasound. Incidental findings of widespread endometriosis and adhesions are often noted with laparoscopic appendectomy and cholecystectomy. Flexible sigmoidoscopy and colonoscopy findings obstructing or narrowing the patency of the colon may arouse suspicion of pathology in surrounding structures.

Pelvic Masses

There are several other situations and pelvic structures that may be confused as a gynecological mass or pathology. It is important for the sonographer to find the origin of these other non-gynecological structures. If this is not possible, then documentation of normal appearing gynecological and non-gynecological structure is helpful as a process of elimination. Diverticula in the colon, abscessed colon, colonic mass, inflammatory bowel disease, and stool may be confused with a gynecologic mass. Appendicitis, urinary bladder distention, urinary diverticula, and ureter stone or dilation also needs to be differentiated from gynecologic pelvic structures.

Vaginal Pathology

An imperforate hymen is the most common vaginal-outflow obstruction anomaly in females. It may be diagnosed from the neonatal period through adolescence. It usually presents as a bulging vaginal mass, which is due to retained vaginal secretions. Ultrasound or MRI is the preferred definitive diagnosis when this is present versus aspiration. A transverse vaginal septum may also be present independently or with an imperforate hymen. Gartner's duct cysts are remnants, in the vaginal wall, of fetal development. If they remain after birth, they can retain fluid and develop mass-effect and infection. Nabothian cysts are common benign cystic masses of the cervix. They can be visualized clinically when performing a speculum examination, or sonographically. Cervical cancer is a pathology that may be seen at the cervix; however, it is rarely detected by sonography. Pap smear is the screening/diagnosis method of choice for cervical carcinoma.

Uterine Malformations

All are uterine malformations that develop when the Müllerian ducts do not fuse together correctly.

- Didelphys uterus – occurs when the Müllerian ducts don't fuse and develop into 2 separate cavities, forming 2 uteruses. They may have an individual or shared cervix and a single or divided vagina.
- Duplex bicollis uterus – two separate uteruses, two cervixes and one vagina.
- Bicornate uterus – two fused uteruses (two uterine horns), one cervix and one vagina (upside down heart).
- Unicornuate uterus – occurs when only one of the Müllerian ducts forms. Often called a "one-sided uterus" or "half-uterus" (banana shape).
- Septated uterus – occurs when the Müllerian ducts fuse, but a partition remains. This septum usually just involves the body of the uterus, but may be seen as a complete partition from the uterus to the cervix and vagina.

Uterine Masses

Leiomyomas

Leiomyomas, more commonly termed uterine fibroids, are the most common benign pelvic mass in females. They usually develop after 30 years of age. The growths arise from the cells that make up the wall layers of the uterus. Patient complaints (increased menstrual flow and pain) and/or a mass palpated on pelvic exam prompts further evaluation. Ultrasound is diagnostic. Fibroids arising from the outer uterine layer may grow to a size larger than the uterus itself. Growth and development of leiomyomas appear to be the result of increased estrogen levels. Treatment options include: watchful waiting, medications, hysteroscopy, myomectomy, or hysterectomy.

Leiomyosarcoma and Adenomyosis

Leiomyosarcoma of the uterus is an extremely rare cancer that arises from the smooth muscle cells of the myometrium of the uterine wall. Its prognosis is poor. The presence of uterine fibroids, even if severe, does not predispose a woman to the development of leiomyosarcoma. Adenomyosis is more commonly termed endometriosis. It is a noncancerous condition in which the cells that make up the layer of the inner uterus, endometrium, grow outside of the uterus. This can cause pain, menstrual irregularities and decreased fertility. The condition is diagnosed by patient history, physical exam, and usually confirmed with transvaginal ultrasound or laparoscopy.

Endometrial Pathology

Endometrioid, Clear Cell Tumors, Brenner Tumors

Endometrioid tumors, clear cell tumors and transitional cell or Brenner tumors are all a type of surface epithelial-stromal tumor. They are far less prevalent than the others in the class (serous and mucinous cystadenomas). Sonographically, they are difficult to differentiate from each other. Endometrioid ovarian tumors are unilateral or bilateral arising from endometrial cells, often making it difficult to determine if this is a primary endometrioid ovarian tumor or from secondary endometrium cancer. Clear cell ovarian tumors have a very poor prognosis. They are unilateral or bilateral and arise from mesonephric tissue. Often endometriosis is in coexistence when a clear cell tumor is diagnosed. Brenner or transitional cell tumors are benign, small and usually unilateral. Sonographically, they are often solid with well-defined borders.

Endometritis

Endometritis is an infection of the endometrial lining. Arguably, the terminology is incorrect, as infection can extend beyond the boundaries of the endometrium. In this case, the term metritis is more descriptive, and includes endometrial, myometrial and parametrial infection. Endometritis may arise after cesarean section, PID or dilation and curettage procedures. On sonography, the endometrial layer is irregular and thickened. Furthermore, metritis may be observed on sonography with uterine air bubbles and debris within the endometrium. However, sonographic finding may also be normal and debris may be mistaken for retained products of conception or an intrauterine hematoma.

Endometrial Hyperplasia

Endometrial hyperplasia is the result of thickening of the endometrial lining, without its cyclical sloughing. The increasing thickness is the result of prolonged and abnormal estrogen stimulation. This can occur when the body produces too much estrogen, when the body doesn't produce enough progesterone to balance estrogen production, conditions such as PCOS with anovulation but continued estrogen production, and certain medications such as estrogen-only hormone therapy and Tamoxifen. Sonograph is helpful in the diagnosis of endometrial hyperplasia, but may not differentiate it from endometrial cancer or polyps. Endometrial hyperplasia is most common in the perimenopausal female.

Endometrial Carcinoma

Endometrial carcinoma is considered an estrogen-dependent cancer. It is most common in the postmenopausal population and accounts for the leading type of female organ cancer in the United States. Endometrial carcinoma should be excluded first in any vaginal bleeding that occurs in a postmenopausal patient. There is a relationship between endometrial hyperplasia and the development of endometrial carcinoma, but it is not clear at what point or for what reason the hyperplastic state turns cancerous. A thickened and irregular end endometrium is present on sonographic evaluation, but this is true with many gynecological conditions. Echogenic tumors and myometrial involvement and irregularity may also be present. These findings may be further evaluated with sonohysterography or hysterosalpingography, but ultimately biopsy is definitive.

Endometrial Adhesions

Endometrial adhesions, synonymous with Asherman syndrome, are secondary to scar tissue formation within the uterus. This is most commonly secondary to aggressive or multiple dilation and curettage procedures, but may also be seen as a result of any pelvic surgery or infection. Asherman syndrome often results in infertility or recurrent miscarriage. Plain sonographic evaluation has limited value in the diagnosis of endometrial adhesions. Sonohysterography and hysteroscopy are more definitive tests, as these will demonstrate a characteristic webbed pattern. Testing is best done during the secretory phase of the menstrual cycle.

Endometriosis

Endometriosis is the growth and development of endometrial cells and tissue outside of the uterus. Endometriosis is seen in women in their 20s and 30s. The exact incidence is unknown, because there may be asymptomatic endometriosis. Diagnosis is often incidental, through other abdominal/pelvic procedures. Although endometriosis can occur almost anywhere, common sites are the ovaries, uterosacral and rectovaginal areas as well as the colon itself. If there is a focal area of endometriosis, it is often termed endometrioma. Endometriomas may be detected on sonography, as they may appear as echoic cysts with debris, fine strands or they may present as a hemorrhagic cyst. Definitive diagnosis is with a combination of laparoscopic and histologic evaluation.

Cervical Pathology

Possible Ultrasound Findings When Assessing the Cervix

Blood or other fluids may be visualized within the cervix (endocervical canal) during an ultrasound evaluation. In addition to fluid, structures such as polyps may also be identified. A cervical polyp is a benign (noncancerous) mass, but it may create symptoms such as abnormal or heavy bleeding. The size and location of these polyps can be determined on ultrasound. Pap smears are the gold standard to determine abnormal cells of the cervix, but ultrasound will often demonstrate masses of the cervix. Cervical cancer is typically a hypoechoic or isoechoic lesion when visualized sonographically, but sometimes the only sign is an enlarged cervix. Ultrasound can also be used to determine if other adjacent structures are involved in the presence of a mass. Color Doppler evaluation may provide useful data pertaining to the vascularity of the tumor.

Ultrasound Appearance of Nabothian Cysts

Nabothian cysts are commonly visualized sonographically within the cervix in women of childbearing ages, after childbirth, or with any disorder that causes inflammation of the cervix. The cervix contains mucus that is produced by the glands located within, and nabothian cysts are produced when these glands become obstructed by the skin that covers them. Ultrasound demonstrates anechoic cysts that are typically very small (often less than 1 cm), and often more than one will be displayed in the cervical region. Color Doppler will not display blood flow within these structures. They do not typically cause symptoms, so surgical intervention is not required unless they become symptomatic and cause pain. Ablation or cryotherapy may be the primary treatment choices when these cysts need to be removed. These cysts can be diagnosed with transvaginal and transabdominal approaches.

Pelvic Inflammatory Disease

PID (Pelvic Inflammatory Disease) is an infection that originates at the cervix and endocervix, often spreading superiorly to involve other pelvic structures. There are many causative organisms, but Chlamydia trachomatis and Neisseria gonorrhea are the most common. Oral contraceptive pills make the mucosa less favorable for PID to develop. Early in the disease, sonographic diagnosis may not be possible but is important to exclude other disorders such as ectopic pregnancy and appendicitis. Later, several characteristic sonographic findings may be present. If the fallopian tubes are affected, the "cogwheel" sign may be present with increased tubal thickening. The tube may also contain fluid and nodular, "beads on a string". Laparoscopy with or without culture is definitive, but not always necessary.

Other Uterine Findings

Sonographic Appearance of a C-Section Scar Defect

Ultrasound is used to evaluate and diagnose a cesarean-section (C-section) scar defect. Ultrasound can help physicians determine the integrity of the scar in patients that have had prior C-sections. Possible defects are important to recognize so that future pregnancy complications do not occur. A transvaginal approach is the preferred method to evaluate C-section scars, and it may be performed with or without saline. To locate the C-section scar, sonographers should evaluate the anterior myometrium of the lower segment of the uterus. The visualization of an echogenic line extending anteriorly from the endometrium is an indication of a C-section scar that is intact. If thinning of the myometrium is observed, it is assumed that the scar is defective. Rupture and the occurrence of an ectopic pregnancy within the scar are also concerns that sonographers should be aware of. One risk of a C-section is the formation of a niche, which is a hypoechoic triangular defect that may be seen with ultrasound interrogation in the area of the incision. This defect may fill with blood, which will give it an anechoic appearance. This may create pain, may interfere with fertility, and may even create defects in a scar that has not already healed.

Leiomyoma and Leiomyosarcoma

Leiomyomas (also referred to as fibroids) are benign tumors that are found in the uterus. Because of their estrogen dependence, these uterine masses are often diagnosed in women in their reproductive years. During pelvic exams, physicians may note an enlarged uterus. Typically, their sonographic appearance is that of a solid, hypoechoic mass(es) that does not demonstrate through transmission. Cystic degeneration may occur the longer the patient has the fibroid(s), and calcifications may be noted. A leiomyosarcoma, on the other hand, is an aggressive, malignant form of uterine cancer that develops from previous leiomyomas. Although they are relatively rare, there is a grim prognosis for patients that are diagnosed with these tumors. Frequently, the only indicator that a uterine mass is a leiomyosarcoma is when the mass appears to undergo accelerated progression in postmenopausal women. When color or power Doppler is used, leiomyosarcomas typically demonstrate increased vascularity. They can be difficult to discern from a fibroid because they also appear hypoechoic without through transmission (unless the leiomyosarcoma has undergone cystic degeneration).

Ovarian Pathology

DES Exposure Malformations

The population that deserves the most consideration for complications and malformations associated with DES exposure are those born between 1940 and 1970. At that time, DES was being given to pregnant women of high-risk pregnancies. It has been determined that fetal exposure to DES not only increases the risk of female organ cancer, but also increases uterine malformation as well. The inferior portion of the uterus, including the cervix, is the area most affected by the DES exposure. The endometrial canal and cervical os are severely narrowed by DES exposure. With this and the less affected fundus of the uterus, sonographic imaging with radiopaque material, often produces a "T" appearance of the endometrial cavity.

Ovarian Cancer

A high-degree of suspicion is important for detection of ovarian cancer in the patient who has abnormal or postmenopausal bleeding, pelvic mass, family history of ovarian cancer, personal history of cancer (especially female organ), and nulliparous women. Both pelvic and transvaginal sonography are recommended. Any adnexal or ovarian mass should be described thoroughly in terms of size and consistency. Cystic ovarian structures, fairly common and normal in a menstruating female, should increase concern in the postmenopausal ovary, especially if they are greater than 10 mm in size. Septations and nodules within an ovarian cyst are also a concerning finding for an ovarian cancer. Low resistive index with Doppler evaluation, of an ovarian mass, also increases concern for ovarian cancer.

Epithelial-Stromal Tumors

Serous cystadenoma is the most common benign ovarian tumor. Cystadenomas are usually unilateral, smaller than mucinous cysts, more likely unilocular with thin but well-defined walls and thin septa. Serous cystadenocarcinoma are the most common ovarian cancer, often involving bilateral ovaries. Sonographically, serous cystadenocarcinoma are also smaller than mucinous cysts. The borders of serous cystadenocarcinoma are irregular and the walls are thick. This carcinoma is highly septated, multilocular and often has internal papillary projections. Cystadenofibroma are similar to the above two adenomas plus fibroids, as they display greater areas of solid tissue on ultrasound.

A mucinous cystadenoma is a benign ovarian tumor, usually unilateral, large (at least 15 cm), and it is not unheard of to have one of these weigh greater than 100 pounds. Ultrasound reveals a simple cyst with thin walls and multilocular septations. The cyst contains a thick, gelatin-like material. Mucinous cystadenocarcinoma is a malignant ovarian tumor that can be unilateral or bilateral, usually found in the menopausal patient. They are large tumors, much like that of the mucinous cystadenoma, but are more likely to rupture. On sonograph these have thick and irregular walls and septations. Mucinous cystadenocarcinomas also contain hypoechoic fluid, often with debris present. If a mucinous cystadenocarcinoma ruptures, it is called pseudomyxoma peritonei. Sonographically, pseudomyxoma peritonei reveals loculated ascites and mass effect. Pseudomyxoma peritonei can also be present from rupture of other mucinous tumors of other organs such as the appendix and bowel.

Cystic Teratoma

Dermoid cysts are a germ cell type tumor. Although they are rare in terms of all types of ovarian tumors, they are the most common ovarian tumor in patients 25 years of age and younger. Dermoid cysts are usually unilateral with a symmetrical shape. Average size is 15 cm but they may be as large as 40 cm. The sonographic appearance of a cystic teratoma is highly varied. Often times, the mass will contain material with hair, fat, teeth, bone, and cartilage-like material. Sonographically, the dermoid cyst can appear either solid or cystic with a great deal of shadowing. Approximately 70% of ovarian dermoid cysts are benign.

Struma Ovarii and Teratomas

Struma ovarii are germ cell tumors that are usually benign, composed of mature thyroid-like tissue. As a result, struma ovarii produce thyroid hormone. They are hard to differentiate, sonographically, from a cystic teratoma. Mature solid teratomas are germ cell tumors that sonographically appear solid. They are slow growing and more common between the ages of 10 and 20 years. Immature teratomas are malignant germ cell tumors primarily affecting adolescents. Sonographically, immature teratomas appear solid but contain many tiny cysts and highly echogenic. Immature teratomas grow rapidly are usually unilateral.

Granulosa Cell and Sertoli-Leydig Tumors

Granulosa cell tumors arise from the gonadal stromal cells. They are functional, meaning they produce hormones. These can affect all age groups but are more likely to be benign in older patients, but can lead to endometrial carcinoma in the menopausal patient. Granulosa cell tumors are primarily unilateral. Sertoli-Leydig tumors are more appropriately termed arrhenoblastomas (Sertoli-Leydig tumor of the ovary), as this differentiates them from Sertoli-Leydig tumors of the testes. They arise from gonadal stromal cells. These tumors are an average size of 10 cm and produce male hormone, thus patients with arrhenoblastomas will often demonstrate masculine characteristics.

Dysgerminoma and Yolk Sac Tumors

Dysgerminomas are germ cell tumors, commonly unilateral, malignant, affects those under 30 years of age and are often diagnosed in pregnancy. They are the most common germ cell tumor seen in patients with gonadal dysgenesis. Sonographically monitoring will result in observation of rapid growth and a multilobular textured, solid mass. Yolk sac tumors are germ cell tumors also known as endodermal sinus tumors. They are malignant, affect patients at an average age of 20 years, and are unilateral. Sonographic appearance is usually a solid mass that is encapsulated and has varying shape and size.

Krukenberg's Tumor

Krukenberg's tumor is a term used to describe a secondary ovarian tumor, or a tumor that has metastasized from another organ or site. Metastatic ovarian tumors are largely (80%) from a gastrointestinal (stomach and colon) site. Krukenberg's tumors are often bilateral and contain signet-ring cells. They are a mucinous carcinoma and often infiltrative. Although the term Krukenberg's tumor initially was used to describe metastatic tumors of the ovary from a gastrointestinal source, it is now commonplace to use it to describe ovarian metastatic tumors from all sources including the breast. Krukenberg's tumors represent up to 10% of all ovarian tumors.

Fibromas and Comas

An ovarian fibroma is a type of gonadal stromal cell tumor; however, unlike other tumors in this category, it does not secrete hormones. Ovarian fibromas are often benign. They can vary greatly in size. Sonographically, the ovarian fibroma has smooth and regular borders, solid in appearance and often associated with ascites. An ovarian thecoma is also a gonadal stromal cell tumor that does produce hormone. Ovarian thecomas are benign and mostly unilateral with varying size. Differentiating ovarian thecomas from ovarian fibromas via sonograph is difficult.

Ovarian Carcinoma Screening

Pelvic examination, Pap smear, ultrasound, and tumor marker tests such as CA125 have all been evaluated for ovarian cancer screening. However, none of these individual options or combinations has stepped to the forefront for a variety of reasons: specificity, cost versus benefit ratio, and impact on overall survival rate, and the presence/absence of definitive treatment. Important to all of these is a thorough patient history, as there are several known risk factors for the development of ovarian carcinoma: family history, age >50, nulliparous, history of breast cancer, race, Jewish descent, HRT in postmenopause, and fertility drugs. The CA125 test is erroneous in the fact that it is nonspecific and often positive in premenopausal patient in a number of benign conditions. Furthermore, it does not detect all types of ovarian carcinomas at any age. Currently, if a patient possesses > 2 risk factors, performing a CA125 and sonography is reasonable.

Ovarian Carcinoma

The prevalence of ovarian carcinoma, in the United States, annually is approximately 22,000 diagnosed cases. Of these, over half are fatal. Ovarian carcinoma represents about one-quarter of all female organ cancers and is the fourth leading cause of cancer death among women in the United States. Incidence of malignancy increases proportionately with age. Mortality is highly dependent upon the stage of cancer at the time of diagnosis. In general, for a variety of reasons, those with ovarian carcinoma usually present and are diagnosed later in the disease. The average 5-year survival rate, after diagnosis of ovarian carcinoma, is approximately 42%. Morbidity ranges from chronic pain, abdominal distension, bowel obstruction and multiple gastrointestinal symptoms, as well as numerous self-image and emotional difficulties.

Corpus Luteum Cyst

Corpus luteum cysts are benign cysts, but before diagnosing them, ectopic pregnancy should be ruled-out. The sonographic appearances of corpus luteum cysts are difficult to differentiate from that of the sonographic appearance of an ectopic pregnancy. A corpus luteum cyst forms from hemorrhage into the luteum after ovulation. Average size of a corpus luteum cyst is 4 cm but can be as great as 10 cm. These cysts are commonly seen early in pregnancy, reaching maximal size by 10 weeks of pregnancy. Rupture and spontaneous resolution occur by the end of the first trimester. Sonographic characteristics include: complex to cystic mass, central blood clot, and septations (lacy pattern) within the clot. Corpus luteum cyst and hemorrhagic cyst are often synonymous.

Follicular Ovarian Cysts

Follicular cysts are normal sonographic findings in the menstruating female. Follicles are formed every time the ovary produces an egg. Follicles increase to maximal size at ovulation, and then burst to release the egg. It is when the follicles don't release the egg and continue to grow that we call them follicular cysts. Follicular cysts are greater than 2.5 cm, average about 6-8 cm and can be as big as 20 cm. They usually spontaneously regress over the course of a few menstrual cycles; this can be monitored by ultrasound. If follicular cysts do not shrink to less than 8 cm over the course of monitoring (3-5 cycles), consider further work-up and alternate diagnosis.

Paraovarian Cysts

Paraovarian cysts often form as the result of a Wolffian duct remnant. Paraovarian cysts are benign and fairly common (10% of all pelvic masses. They are found in the broad ligament and do not arise within the ovary. This can often be differentiated with the transvaginal ultrasound and they are often visualized above the fundus. They have the sonographic appearance of a normal cysts but may be hemorrhagic and torsed. Paraovarian cysts are generally less than 5 cm and their size will not fluctuate with the menstrual cycle. However, paraovarian cysts can increase in size and extend into the abdominal cavity, making determination of origin difficult.

Theca Lutein Ovarian Cysts

Theca lutein ovarian cysts are often the result of increased serum human chorionic gonadotropin circulation in the female. They are often comorbid to other conditions such as polycystic ovarian syndrome, gestational trophoblastic disease (hydatidiform mole and choriocarcinomas), multiple gestation, gestational diabetes, and sometimes as a result of some infertility medications. Theca lutein cysts usually spontaneously resolve or rupture by four months; however, they are at increased risk for torsion and hemorrhage. The patient with theca lutein cysts may complain of pelvic pain, dyspareunia, nausea and vomiting. Sonographically, bilateral ovarian enlargement will be present. Ovarian cysts will be multilocular and will also be found in both ovaries.

Dermoid Cyst Confusion

Due to the highly variable appearance of cystic teratomas, they may be easily confused with other conditions on sonographic examination. Of equal concern is the misdiagnosis of dermoid cysts, when in fact another pelvic pathology is present. Other sonographically similar diagnostic possibilities to cystic teratoma include: ectopic pregnancy, distended bowel, fibroids (especially pedunculated), tubo-ovarian abscess, appendicitis, extraovarian lipomatosis, and any cystic mass with echogenic nodules. Furthermore, sonographic findings can appear "normal", thus the importance of the clinical history. Ovarian torsion or hemorrhage can be secondary to the cystic teratoma or independent of it.

Ovarian Torsion

Ovarian torsion is a condition in which the ovarian pedicle rotates on its axis. There may be complete or partial rotation. This is statistically more common in children and adolescence, with the right ovary, and in the presence of another benign adnexal mass. Clinically, ovarian torsion can act a lot like appendicitis. Fifty percent of the time there is a palpable mass. Sonographically ovarian torsion can vary. Imaged appearance is that of an edematous and enlarged ovary, usually greater than 4 cm. 'Classic' sonographic appearance of ovarian torsion is that of a hypoechoic mass surrounded by multiple small follicles. 'Common' sonographic appearance of ovarian torsion is of a completely solid adnexal mass. Doppler studies may reveal complete absence of blood flow to the ovary is torsion is complete or reduced blood flow to the ovary in partial torsion.

Malignant Ovarian Neoplasms

Serous Carcinoma

Of all cancers that stem from the reproductive system, ovarian cancer is the deadliest. This is often because ovarian malignancies are diagnosed in their later stages because patients are typically asymptomatic. There are multiple types of ovarian cancers, the most malignant of which are high-grade serous ovarian carcinomas (HGSOCs), which are of epithelial origin and are responsible for approximately 80% of ovarian cancer fatalities. Patients with HGSOCs are typically postmenopausal and in their sixties when a diagnosis is made. Ultrasound characteristics include ascites and adnexal masses (unilateral or bilateral) that are multilocular and measure greater than or equal to 5 cm with half of them measuring more than 15 cm. When the tumor is larger than 5 cm, it will often have cystic and solid components. It is not unusual to see internal septations. Color and power Doppler will reveal blood flow within these septations and solid portions. However, when tumors are smaller than 5 cm, it is not uncommon to only visualize a solid mass.

Papillary Cystadenocarcinoma

Papillary cystadenocarcinomas are a type of malignant ovarian cancer of epithelial origin that are often diagnosed in patients in their fifth decade of life or who are postmenopausal. This type of ovarian cancer is a subtype of serous tumors and, unfortunately, like other ovarian neoplasms, are diagnosed in late stages because patients do not have any symptoms. Ultrasound findings often include a unilocular or multilocular appearance of the ovary with multiple papillary projections, which are often visualized near the inner walls of the cysts. These projections are often thickened and irregular and typically exhibit blood flow when color or power Doppler is used. These papillary projections or walls of the cysts may display echogenic foci (with or without posterior shadowing).

Other Ovarian Findings

Polycystic Ovary Syndrome

Polycystic ovary syndrome (PCOS) is the most common female hormonal disorder. It is a disorder marked by anovulatory cycles, partially due to the body producing excess androgens. This can be apparent by heavy or irregular menses, increased facial hair growth, insulin resistance, and fertility difficulties. Diagnosis is made with history, physical exam, lab tests, and ultrasound. The sonographic findings of enlarged ovaries and multiple cysts is not independently diagnostic of PCOS. Complications of PCOS are the development of diabetes, hypertension, lipid disorders, infertility, and endometrial cancer. Treatment options include dietary changes, weight-loss and exercise, hormones, fertility drugs, diabetic drugs (to help with insulin resistance), medications to decrease androgen production, and surgery.

Ultrasound is an important tool to help diagnose females with PCOS because not every individual has the classic symptoms of obesity, oligomenorrhea (or amenorrhea), and hirsutism. A transvaginal approach is preferred to evaluate the ovaries to assess the ovarian volume and the number of follicles. It is not uncommon for females with PCOS to have ovaries that are two to five times their normal size with a volume measuring more than 10 cc (operators should, however, make sure that dominant follicles or corpus luteal cysts are not present when measuring the volume). The number of follicles in each ovary should also be observed, and, in cases of PCOS, it is greater than or equal to 20 follicles. Evaluating the number and size of follicles is the most important criterion in reaching a diagnosis.

Peritoneal Inclusion Cysts

Peritoneal inclusion cysts are more likely to be seen in females with a history of pelvic inflammatory disease, multiple pelvic adhesions, and endometriosis. These develop from fluid produced by the ovaries, which does not absorb normally due to the thickened peritoneum. This fluid becomes entrapped within the fibrotic network, causing the cyst. This is not an ovarian cyst. Clinically and sonographically it is difficult, if not impossible, to differentiate from a paraovarian cyst. A thick layer of mesothelial cells lines peritoneal inclusion cysts. Inclusion cysts can be as large as 20 cm in size. Peritoneal inclusion cysts are synonymous with: benign encysted fluid and benign cystic mesothelioma.

Using Ultrasound to Assess and Diagnose PID

Pelvic inflammatory disease (PID) is a condition of the female reproductive system that stems from unresolved or untreated sexually transmitted infections such as gonorrhea or chlamydia. For symptomatic women, pelvic pain, fever, vaginal discharge, and painful urination or intercourse are often reported. Early on, the cervix and endometrium are affected, but as the infection advances it will also affect the fallopian tubes and ovaries. Ultrasound can offer quick diagnostic results and can be done either transabdominally (in cases in which the patient is experiencing a great deal of pain) or transvaginally (preferred). Depending on the extent of the disease, ultrasound findings will typically include dilated fallopian tubes with thick walls. Incomplete septa represent the kinking of these structures, and echogenic material may be present within cases of a pyosalpinx. Adnexal masses may be present, and the ovaries may be difficult to discern when an abscess has formed. Ascites may also be visualized. Color or power Doppler will often show an increase of vascularity of these structures.

Endometritis

Endometritis is a medical term for the inflammation of the endometrium, which is the inner lining of the uterus. This may be the result of bacteria that has entered the vagina and moved into the endometrium via the cervix as part of a PID. Patients also present with cases of endometritis after childbirth or an abortion, and they often experience fever, pelvic pain, and vaginal discharge. Ultrasound imaging is often used because patients that have a tubo-ovarian abscess or retained products of conception may also present with the same symptoms. Typical sonographic findings of endometritis are typically a thickened endometrium with the presence of fluid or taking on a more hyperechoic appearance when gas is present. It should be noted that gas may be present for approximately three weeks after delivery. In cases of endometrial inflammation, it may be difficult to discern the endometrium from the myometrium. Overall, the uterus may be enlarged.

Pyosalpinx

Salpingitis is a unilateral or bilateral inflammation of the fallopian tube. It is the result of acute or chronic PID. When the fallopian tube becomes distended with pus due to the bacteria within, it is referred to as a pyosalpinx. Transvaginal ultrasound is a useful tool to evaluate patients with this condition, but sonographers should be aware that patients may experience considerable tenderness due to the inflammation. Ultrasound findings include a tortuous adnexal mass that is located adjacent to the ovary. This mass may have partial internal septations due to the kinks of the tube and may display low-level internal echoes. This sonographic finding may help distinguish a hydrosalpinx (filled with clear fluid) from a pyosalpinx.

Tubo-Ovarian Abscess

The quick and accurate diagnosis of a tubo-ovarian abscess is imperative because these patients are often extremely sick; treatment includes antibiotics, surgery, and/or drainage of the abscess (which may be done under ultrasound guidance). During a transvaginal ultrasound, the patient's lower abdomen may be extremely tender because the cause of a tubo-ovarian abscess is PID that was not treated. The ultrasound appearance of a tubo-ovarian abscess may include unilateral or bilateral complex adnexal masses where it is difficult to discern the ovary. A "cogwheel" sign is often present, which represents a cross section of an inflamed tube with walls that are thickened. The walls often measure greater than or equal to 5 mm. The fallopian tubes are often folded and will appear as multiple, partial septa. Low-level echoes may be present in the dilated tube. Free fluid may also be present in the posterior cul-de-sac. Color and power Doppler interrogation of the abscess will demonstrate peripheral blood flow of the mass as well as within the septa. A 3D ultrasound scan can also be performed to gain a better understanding of the extent of the pathology.

Intrauterine Contraceptive Device (IUCD) Location

Transvaginal ultrasound can be used to determine the location of an intrauterine contraceptive device (IUCD). A sagittal view of the uterus should be performed with the stem of the IUCD visualized as a highly reflective linear structure within the endometrial canal that casts a posterior shadow. This device should be within the fundus of the uterus when positioned in the correct location. Transverse imaging should also be used to confirm that the endometrium is not separate from the IUCD. If it is not present in the upper portion of the endometrial canal, the sonographer should evaluate the lower portion of the uterus and the cervix. If the IUCD is still not seen, the myometrium should be evaluated to determine embedment (migration into the myometrium) versus perforation (migration outside of the uterus). If the IUCD is not visualized sonographically within the uterus, an abdominal radiograph may be ordered to identify its location. Sonographers may also use 3D applications to confirm the location of the IUCD in the coronal plane, which will allow the stem and arms to be imaged concurrently.

Obstetrics - First Trimester

Normal Anatomy and Physiology

General Uses of Sonography

Sonography may be used in obstetrical practice to assist in diagnosis of pregnancy. Ultrasound can detect the gestational sac at about 5 weeks or when corresponding beta-hCG levels are 5000 mIU/ml. Ultrasound serves as the most accurate determination of gestational age; this is often done in the late first trimester to early second trimester. Doppler devices are used to monitor fetal heart activity throughout pregnancy. Ultrasound is also the most accurate tool in assessing fetal growth and activity. It may also be used to assess fetal abnormalities. Sonography can indirectly help assess fetal maturity, but this is not the most accurate or first-line test for fetal maturity assessment.

Fertilization to Embryo Development

Fertilization occurs when a female oocyte unites with a male sperm cell. Together, these form a zygote that implants itself into the female endometrium. Implantation of the zygote is the official beginning of pregnancy. The zygote goes through mitotic divisions and forms the placenta, umbilical cord, and eventually the embryo. The embryonic phase starts at about week 3 and continues through week 8. Early in the embryonic phase, the growth centers on what will be the spine and spinal cord. By week 6, the embryo produces chemicals to cease the menstrual cycle. Brain activity can be noted at this time and the heart beat starts. Organogenesis begins, limb buds form and the head is over half of the mass of the embryo. By week 8 of embryogenesis, the embryo is capable or movement, eyes are forming and blood type develops. At the end of the 8th week, the embryo state is complete and moves into the fetal stage.

Assessment in the First Trimester

American Institute of Ultrasound in Medicine guidelines for sonography in the first trimester includes use of real-time equipment. The minimum necessary approach should be performed. If the transabdominal approach gathers accurate and appropriate information, then the transvaginal approach does not need to be completed, and vice versa. Both approaches may be needed. Presence, location, and content of gestational sac should be noted. If applicable, crown rump measurements should be included versus gestational sac measurements; these allow for more accurate gestational age determinations. An embryo or yolk sac must be present before noting the presence of a gestational sac. Note cardiac motion if crown rump is at least 5 mm. Determination of fetal number can only be based on embryo number, not on multiple sac-like structures. Document your evaluation and the appearance of all the surrounding structures including adnexa and cul-de-sacs.

Timing of Obstetrical Sonogram

The optimal timing of the obstetric sonograph is dependent on the purpose that is hopes to achieve. If it is strictly gestational age that is sought, the earlier the sonograph can be performed and the measurements taken, the better. Gestational age determination is most accurate in the first trimester. If fetal monitoring, development, and screening for anomalies are the goal of sonography, then early second trimester sonography is preferred. Most fetal images can be viewed with great detail, and anomalies detected by 18 weeks of gestation. If only one ultrasound can be performed, selecting a time in between these two ideals is suggested. A single ultrasound between the 12th and 16th weeks is acceptable and widely used.

Determination of Pregnancy

The gestational sac can be viewed with sonography as early as 4 weeks. This is the first sonographic evidence of pregnancy. Gestational sac diameter may be measured and correlated with gestational age initially, but after 8 gestational weeks, this is no longer used. The diameter of the gestational sac at 5 weeks is usually about 5 mm. The yolk sac can be viewed at about 5 weeks with sonography. The presence of the yolk sac on sonogram is the first sign of embryonic structure or formation. It is located between the chorion and the amnion and its measurements are recorded along with those of the gestational sac.

Gestational Age

Determining an accurate gestational age is important for obstetrical management and planning. It is also imperative for monitoring fetal development and normalcy. If an anomaly is found, it is important to know if this is a "normal variant" or a true concern based on gestational age. Accurate gestational age determination is important for scheduling and interpreting routine obstetrical tests. If the need for invasive obstetrical testing arises, such as amniocentesis and chorionic villus sampling, correct timing and appropriate windows are imperative. Gestational age determination allows for more accurate estimation of delivery, whether that be spontaneous or a planned cesarean delivery. If a serious abnormality is discovered, accurate gestational age is important in helping the mother determine her options for management.

The gestational age refers to the time since conception. Conception refers to the event and time at which the blastocyte implants itself into the endometrium. The gestational age is usually two weeks later than the first day of the last menstrual period. The term gestational age is often used interchangeably with menstrual age, even though the two terms or definitions technically differ by two weeks. Menstrual age is the time from the first day of the last menstrual period. This is the more commonly used age determinant, although inaccurate patient reporting limits this method.

Since there are limitations to obtaining accurate gestational or menstrual age from the patient (irregular menstrual cycles and inaccurate recall), sonography has become the mainstay and most accurate determinant of gestational age. In the first trimester, the most accurate sonographic gestational age determinants are crown-rump length and biparietal diameter. These can be used individually or in combination. The crown-rump length may be easier to determine initially. The head circumference, femur length, and abdominal circumference may also support sonographic gestational age determinations. If sonography is performed after the first trimester, its accuracy for determining gestational age declines. In this case, all of the above measurements plus last menstrual period should be used to determine the most likely gestational age.

Accuracy of Gestational Age

Sonographic first trimester gestational age determination is the most accurate and widely used. Even if second and third trimester sonographic measurements of crown-rump, biparietal, head circumference, and femur length suggest a different gestational age, the earliest sonographic measurements will be deferred to for gestational age determinants. The gestational age is either determined by chorionic sac diameter when this is between 2 mm and 14 mm, or by the earliest crown-rump measurement. Although first trimester measurements are preferable is gestational age determination, accuracy can still be maintained up to 20 weeks.

Gestational Sac Findings

Gestational sac is synonymous with chorionic sac. The earliest sonographically visualized gestational sac is about 4.5 weeks gestation. It is viewed as a small, well-defined echogenic ring with a hypoechoic center. The horizontal line below the gestational sac is the endometrial cavity; the appearance of this is called the intradecidual sign. This must be present to identify a true intrauterine gestational sac. The gestational sac may be visualized at 2 mm diameter with transvaginal technique. With transabdominal technique, the gestational sac may not be apparent until it is at least 5 mm diameter. The gestational sac should be visualized near the fundus of the uterus. Measurements of the gestational sac (length, width and depth) are highly correlated with HCG levels and gestational age up to 8 weeks.

Intradecidual and Double Decidual Sign

The main value of the sonographic appearance of the intradecidual sign is to exclude the possibility of an ectopic pregnancy. The intradecidual sign is defined as the presence of a fluid collection surrounded by an echogenic border that is located directly adjacent to the central endometrial cavity. This is the earliest sonographic sign of pregnancy and should be differentiated from a similar described finding located within the central endometrial cavity that would indicate a pseudogestational sac or ectopic pregnancy. The double decidual sign may first be observed at 5.5 weeks of a normal intrauterine pregnancy. It is composed of the decidua vera and decidua capsularis that form an echogenic ring. This will not be present in an ectopic pregnancy.

Decidual Thickening Findings

Decidual thickening is literally a thickening of the endometrium at the site of implantation. This has an echogenic appearance on sonography and may actually be the earliest sonographic sign of pregnancy. However, it is rare to define pregnancy solely on this finding. The yolk sac may be identified within the gestational sac as early as 5 weeks, via transvaginal imaging. The presence of a yolk sac is the truest determination of a valid gestational sac. The yolk sac is echogenic and sphere shaped. The yolk sac is usually positioned at a border of the gestational sac.

Double Bleb Sign

The double bleb sign is a sonographic finding seen from about 5.5 weeks up to 7 weeks gestation. Two adjacent, circular shapes with echogenic outer borders mark this sign. These represent the yolk sac and the amniotic sac. Lying in between these "blebs" is a small echogenic embryo. This follows that the embryo may first be visualized by ultrasound at about 5 weeks. If imaging this early, the transvaginal approach is recommended and may be the only means of viewing the 1-2 mm embryo at this stage. Embryo heart movements may be seen as early as 5 weeks, but is best recorded when the embryo itself is at least 5 mm and the gestational sac 16 mm.

Chorionic Sac

Gestational dates can be estimated with a great degree of accuracy based on sonographic visualization of the gestational or chorionic sac. This is true regardless of the actual gestational sac measurements and is secondary to the fact that there is very little size variability in the first 8 gestational weeks. Sonographic viewing of only the gestational sac suggests a gestational age of 5 weeks. Sonographic visualization of the gestational sac plus yolk sac suggests a gestational age of 5 weeks and 5 days. Sonographic imaging of the chorionic sac plus yolk sac plus a small embryo suggests a gestational age of 6 weeks.

Decidua Basalis, Capsularis, Vera, and Parietalis

The decidua basalis is the term used to describe the maternal endometrium that is located directly inferior to the fetal placenta. This is the site in the inner uterine wall, where implantation occurs. Decidua basalis is synonymous with decidua serotina. Decidua capsularis may also be known as decidua reflexa. The decidua capsularis is a thin portion of endometrium that has direct contact with the chorionic villi. The decidua vera and decidua parietalis are used interchangeably and describe all other areas of the endometrial lining that are not in contact with the chorion.

Mistaken Normal Fetal Structures

Along with nuchal translucency measurements, a few other normal fetal structures can be mistaken for abnormalities. Defective brain or bony cranial vault development cannot be determined or diagnosed with first trimester sonography. Sonography of anencephaly (or lack-thereof) in the first trimester is not predictive of actual development later. Diagnosis of herniation has been made mistakenly; it is normal for bowel to be herniated into the umbilical cord base between 8-13 weeks. This regresses by week 14. Between weeks 7 and 9, a posterior fossa cystic mass may be misdiagnosed. This is a normal finding as the fourth ventricle develops (rhombencephalon).

Gestational Ages to Discern Various Bones of Extremities

When an ultrasound is performed around the 8th week in utero, the sonographer may see tiny limbs extending from the body of the embryo. Movement of the limbs will be seen after 11 weeks because the long bones of the skeleton are easily seen by this stage because ossification has taken place. After 13 weeks, the sonographer may use various biometric measurements instead of the CRL to determine the gestational age. One such bone that is often used in fetal measurements is the femur length. The femur (thigh bone) can often be visualized after 9 weeks, and it is one parameter used to estimate fetal age by 14 weeks. The humerus (upper arm bone) can be visualized after 9 weeks, and it may also be used to determine gestational age. The bones of the forearm (radius and ulna) are seen around 10 weeks, with the phalanges more readily seen after 11 weeks. The bones of the lower leg (tibia and fibula) are also visualized well after 10 weeks with the digits of the foot seen after 11 weeks.

Length of the Embryonic Pole by the End of the 10th Week

During human development, weeks 6 through 10 are considered to be the embryonic period. In this stage, the proportions and the shape of the embryo are considerably altered. At the beginning of this stage, the head is disproportionate, and it consumes nearly half of the entire embryonic pole. By the end of the embryonic period, the head becomes more proportionate with the rest of the crown-rump length (CRL). The CRL will measure about 30 mm near the end of this period. With the exception of the heart, the other organ systems are present, but they are not yet fully functional by the end of the 10th week. It is important to note that the gastrointestinal organs develop quickly, and the intestines are temporarily displaced within the umbilical cord. This makes the GI tract a common site for anomalies to occur.

Obstetrical Ultrasound Between 10 and 14 Weeks of Gestation

An ultrasound performed between 10 and 14 weeks of gestation should include the presence (and number) of a fetus; sonographers should also check for movement of the fetus. Cardiac activity should also be documented by using a video clip in addition to calculating the heart rate. Today's ultrasound systems provide excellent resolution compared with machines used in the past, and many anatomical structures can be visualized and measured to provide an estimated due date. Many labs still use the crown-rump length (CRL) measurement during this time to provide an accurate estimate of gestational age, especially between 10 and 13 weeks. CRL is a measurement of the embryo or fetus from the top of the head to the bottom of the buttocks. This measurement does not include the lower extremities, and it is the most accurate for dates as long as the measurement is performed correctly. If a CRL measurement is provided in the first trimester of pregnancy, the due date should not be changed later on.

Structures of the Brain Visualized with Ultrasound Between 10 and 14 Weeks of Gestation

The sonographer should be able to see the fetal head by 12 weeks of gestation, and with the resolution of today's machines, many structures of the central nervous system should be seen by the end of the 14th week. A measurement of the nuchal translucency (NT) is often performed between weeks 10 and 14, and it is taken in the posterior portion of the fetal neck to help determine the possibility of chromosomal abnormalities. The sonographer must make sure that the NT is evaluated when the neck of the fetus is in a neutral position and that the calipers are placed correctly on the inside portions. A measurement greater than or equal to 3 mm is considered abnormal. The cerebral hemispheres, cerebellum, ventricles, thalami, and brain stem are visible by 12 weeks. The fetal face can be seen, with the facial profile by 13 weeks. Sonographers should check for the presence of these intracranial structures so that anencephaly can be ruled out. In this condition, the majority of the brain and skull are missing, but usually the fetus has orbits and facial structures.

Appearance of Abdomen and Pelvis in Scan Done Between 10 and 14 Weeks of Gestation

The fetal stomach will be visualized by 13 weeks of gestation as a sonolucent "bubble" in the left upper quadrant. Sonographers should remember that the midgut extends into the umbilical cord and returns between 10 and 12 weeks. Fetuses scanned after 12 weeks may not display any of the aforementioned herniation because the midgut has likely already returned to the abdomen. Organs of the urinary system may be seen at 12 weeks. The kidneys are often visualized in a transverse plane located on both sides of the spine. The echogenicity of the kidneys tends to increase as the pregnancy progresses due to the amount of perinephric fat. The renal pyramids may be visualized as anechoic areas within the middle portion of the kidneys. The urinary bladder can often be visualized as a small anechoic structure that will change in size as the bladder fills. If the ultrasound user does not see the bladder at the beginning of the scan, it should be reevaluated at the end, especially in the second trimester to help determine renal function. The umbilical cord insertion may be visualized as well, especially during TVUS by 11 weeks.

Multiple Gestations

Zygosity and Chorionicity

Zygosity refers to the number of fertilized ova that a multiple birth fetus develops from. Monozygotic refers to multiple fetuses developing from a single ovum. Trizygotic refers to multiple fetuses developing from three separate eggs. Monozygotic twins are also known as "identical twins" because they arise from same fertilized egg and share similar genetic material. Dizygotic, and higher, are also known as "fraternal" and do not share the same genetic structure. For example, when delivering dizygotes one may be male, and the other female; one with brown hair, and the other with blonde hair. Chorionicity basically refers to the number of placentas present in a pregnancy. A dichorionic pregnancy will have two placentas; a trichorionic pregnancy will have three placentas and etc. Both descriptors are necessary to determine pregnancy management and identify possible complications. A monochorionic pregnancy, of any zygosity, increases the likelihood of twin-to-twin transfusion syndrome and other complications.

Multiple Gestation Factors

Several factors contribute to the increased likelihood of multiple gestation. Increased maternal age, increasing use of fertility treatment medications, and increased in vitro fertilization are responsible for the overall increased incidence of multiple births. The incidence is approximately 1 in every 80 births. Increased maternal parity is also responsible for the increased likelihood of multiple gestation, especially if this number is greater than 6. There is a significantly increased incidence of dizygotic twins in certain African countries. A positive maternal family history of dizygotic twins increases the chance for multiple gestation. Paternal family history and race do not seem to contribute to increased incidence of multiple gestation. Monozygotic twinning also seems to be independent of any incidence variability.

Twins or Multiples Identification

First trimester sonography is preferred for the most accurate assessment of chorionicity and amnionicity. Chorionicity can be determined slightly earlier at five weeks gestation. Sonographic determination of amnionicity is optimal after the 8th gestational week. Both chorionicity and amnionicity determinations are optimal prior to ten weeks of gestation. Identification of chorionicity and amnionicity requires diligent sonographic assessment of the number of gestational sacs/yolk sacs and the number of amniotic sacs. Furthermore, determination of the number of embryonic heartbeats within each gestational sac will correlate directly with each other.

Amnionicity

Amnionicity describes the number of amniotic sacs in multiple gestations. However, amnionicity is not an independent description and is used alongside zygosity and chorionicity. The importance of these descriptors becomes especially important in identifying possible multiple gestational complications. For example, a monochorionic-monoamniotic twin pregnancy is one in which two fetuses are within the same amniotic cavity and share a single placenta. This situation increases the likelihood of umbilical cord entanglement, increasing the risk for fetal mortality. Amnionicity is highly correlated in a one to one ratio with the number of yolk sacs present.

Criteria for Amnionicity and Chorionicity

The sonographic criteria for amnionicity and chorionicity become more difficult in the second and third trimester; furthermore, the criteria are different than the same determinations in the first trimester. Fetal gender should be determined at this stage. The number of placenta indicates the chorionicity; however, fused and single placentas are difficult to evaluate. The interfetal membrane should be sonographically documented with the presence of a 'Lambda' or 'twin peak' sign. The interfetal membrane should be further described in terms of number of layers and thickness. Thick membranes are between 1 and 2 mm and a thin membrane is less than 1 mm. However, the membrane naturally decreases in thickness with pregnancy progression so measurements of membrane thickness are only useful before 26 weeks of gestation.

Normal Twin Fetal Growth

Fetal growth in twin gestations should be similar to that of the single pregnancy growth parameters in the first and second trimesters. At about the third trimester is when we see the separation of growth parameters of singleton versus twin growth curves. In the third trimester the twins will still have steady growth but it will be much slower than that of a single pregnancy. Slight variation in crown-rump length (less than 5 days difference) is acceptable in the first trimester. Fetal weights should also be within 20% of each other; anything greater incurs greater risk for fetal complications. Theoretically, growth of monozygote twins should be similar and dizygotes may display slightly more variation.

Abnormalities and Complications

Gestational Trophoblastic Disorder

Gestational trophoblastic disorder, also known as choriocarcinoma, describes a group of malignant uterine cancers that develop after pregnancy, abortion, or miscarriage. Gestational trophoblastic disorder usually metastasizes readily and widely. Despite the aggressive nature, prognosis is good with a cure rate of up to 95%. After conception, placental growth develops rapidly and does not support the growth and development of a fetus, but instead a tumor. This is termed a molar pregnancy or hydatidiform, which half of the time precedes choriocarcinomas. Sonography may suspect the presence of a choriocarcinoma in the absence of a fetal heartbeat or visualization of cystic structures within enlarged and edematous chorionic villi.

Ectopic Pregnancy

An ectopic pregnancy is one that results in the fertilized egg and sperm unit implanting anywhere outside of the uterine cavity. Some causes of ectopic pregnancy include: previous ectopic pregnancy, PID, abortion, adhesions, endometriosis, pelvic tumors, and use of oral contraceptives (in some cases). Ectopic pregnancy is not compatible with fetal development, and if undetected places the mother at risk. Some studies report incidence as great as one ectopic pregnancy for every 66 intrauterine pregnancies. This is thought to be due to increasing incidence of PID. Despite increasing rates of ectopic pregnancy, maternal mortality rates have been significantly reduced due to earlier diagnostic capabilities. Clinically, ectopic may present as bleeding, pain, a palpable pelvic mass, fever, tenesmus, referred pains to the shoulders, and syncope. Maintain a high index of suspicion, as these symptoms are shared by many other disorders.

Quantitative beta-hCG serum level monitoring is often the first clue that a pregnancy is not progressing normally and also may raise the first suspicion for the diagnosis of ectopic pregnancy. This is true because the physical signs and symptoms may not always be apparent early on or may be mild in their presentation. In normal pregnancy, serum beta-hCG levels should increase by about 66% every 48 hours. If beta-hCG levels are not increasing as expected, ectopic pregnancy should be suspected. To further the diagnosis, sonography is primarily used to "rule-out" intrauterine pregnancy. Sonography does not always image extrauterine pregnancy, but may image findings that increase the possibility. By the time the serum beta-hCG levels reach 1500 mIU/ml, transvaginal ultrasound should be able to identify an intrauterine pregnancy. For transabdominal technique to view an intrauterine pregnancy, serum beta-hCG levels need to be at least 5000 mIU/ml.

The sonographic appearance of a cystic sac viewed within the endometrium may in fact represent a pseudogestational sac of ectopic pregnancy. However, this small cystic endometrial sac may also represent a decidual cyst or a very early but normal intrauterine pregnancy/gestational sac. The double sac sign is helpful in diagnosing an early pregnancy, but does not absolutely eliminate the possibility of ectopic pregnancy. Even with the appearance of an intrauterine yolk sac and embryo, it is important to evaluate the adnexa. A heterotopic pregnancy may exist in which a normal intrauterine gestation and an abnormal extrauterine gestation coexist. It is often recommended to start with the transabdominal sonograph, as this often allows for better viewing of adnexa and extrauterine structures. Follow this technique with transvaginal technique for better uterine and endometrium viewing.

Sonography may be helpful in identifying the location of the ectopic pregnancy; however, Laparoscopy remains the gold standard. The highest percentages of ectopic pregnancies occur in the fallopian tube. This is why one will often hear the terms ectopic and tubal pregnancy used interchangeably, although this is not entirely accurate. About 5% of ectopic pregnancies occur in the fimbria (the very distal, finger-like projections of the fallopian tubes). Approximately 1-2% of ectopic pregnancies may occur at an abdominal source. Less than 1% occur in the cervix and ovary. Of the approximated 95% of ectopic pregnancies occurring in the fallopian tube, 78% of those occur in the distal most portion or ampullary.

Sonographic findings for ectopic pregnancy are largely nonspecific or exclusionary. In fact, about one quarter of patients with ectopic pregnancy will have a normal pelvic and transvaginal sonogram. Probably the most definitive sonographic finding of ectopic pregnancy would be visualization of an adnexal ring and yolk sac with cardiac activity anywhere outside of the intrauterine cavity. Any patient with a positive serum beta-HCG, sonographic evidence of fluid in the pelvis, an adnexal mass, or with no sonographic evidence of intrauterine pregnancy need to be followed closely. Monitoring should at least include repeat beta-hCG levels and sonography every 48 hours.

Fetal Demise Diagnosis

Fetal demise is primarily diagnosed by inability to obtain a fetal heartbeat. Whether through sonographic monitoring or fetal stress testing, lack of fetal heart tones is equivalent to fetal death. Other sonographic findings may include a cystic and degenerating placenta, edematous findings (almost anywhere), poorly defined abdominal organs, and a positive Spaulding sign, which is a finding of overlapping skull bones. Fetal demise is diagnosed before the fetus and conceptus are extracted from the mother. If fetal death occurs prior to 20 gestational weeks, it is considered early. Intermediate fetal demise is diagnosed if the criteria are met between gestational weeks 21 and 28. If fetal death occurs after 28 gestational weeks it is termed late fetal demise.

Other Diagnoses

Lithopedion, also known as 'stone baby', describes a rare condition in which fetal tissue becomes calcified and too large to be reabsorbed by the maternal body. This is more likely to be seen after an ectopic pregnancy.

Infarction describes any condition or location in which there is a sudden (or prolonged) disruption of blood flow (arterial or venous) to a tissue or organ structure. Infarction then results in cell, tissue, or organ death of the structure to which blood supply is compromised.

Exophthalmos describes a congenital or acquired condition in which there is a unilateral or bilateral increased protuberance of the eyeball(s).

Moles

Classic hydatidiform mole, also known as complete hydatidiform or complete mole is a condition only seen in pregnancy. It is caused when either a single haploid sperm or a 2 normal sperm fertilize an egg that does not contain a nucleus. This results in edema of the chorionic villi and an increased number of trophoblastic cells. The incidence of hydatidiform mole (type unspecified) in the US is about 1 in 1000 pregnancies. It is also an incidental finding in as many as 1 in 600 abortions. The incidence in Asian countries is 15 times that of the US for reasons unknown. Approximately 15% of those with complete mole have uterine involvement and about 4% develop metastasis. Risk of developing complete hydatidiform mole is highest with teenage pregnancy and 7-fold with pregnancy greater than age 40.

With the increasing use and availability of obstetrical sonography, complete hydatidiform mole may be diagnosed early before severe maternal symptoms develop. Possible maternal symptoms of complete mole include: vaginal bleeding, hyperemesis, preeclampsia, and hyperthyroidism. Sonographically, uterine enlargement that is greater than expected for gestational age is a classic sign. The fetus is not visible in a complete mole. The echogenic placenta will appear enlarged and cystic. The sonographic term, "bunch of grapes" is often used to describe this finding. In almost half of the cases of complete mole, bilateral theca-lutein ovarian cysts are present. Both ovaries usually appear enlarged with septated cysts.

Partial hydatidiform moles occur when a haploid egg is fertilized by either 2 normal sperm or from one abnormal diploid sperm. The sonographic findings are essentially the same as in complete hydatidiform mole, but less severe. In addition to the classic sonographic findings of molar pregnancy, there is the presence of a fetus or fetal erythrocytes. Furthermore, partial hydatidiform is not readily detectable via sonography in early pregnancy. Often times, the pregnancy appears to be developing normally and sonographic evidence of partial hydatidiform is not present until late second trimester. Those with a partial mole will not develop choriocarcinoma, but 4% will develop persistent nonmetastatic trophoblastic disease that will require chemotherapy. Symptoms of partial mole are similar to those of an incomplete or missed abortion. Vaginal bleeding is usually present and fetal heart tones are not.

There are three situations that may sonographically appear similar to a partial hydatidiform molar pregnancy, and that must be differentiated from this condition. The first situation is a twin pregnancy in which there is one normal twin with a healthy placenta and the presence of a complete or classic hydatidiform mole. The second condition is that of fetal demise. The placental degeneration that takes place after a fetal demise can sonographically be similar to the "bunch of grapes" appearance seen in a molar pregnancy. Chromosomal testing may be necessary to differentiate this situation. Finally, a fetus with Beckwith-Wiedemann syndrome can mimic sonographic findings in partial mole pregnancies. With Beckwith-Wiedemann syndrome, fetal growth restriction will not be observed and fetal anomalies associated with the syndrome will be sonographically evident.

Invasive hydatidiform mole or chorioadenoma destruens is a gestational disease of the trophoblastic cells. Invasive hydatidiform mole occurs when a partial or classic hydatidiform mole grows into the muscular uterine wall. Invasive hydatidiform may develop in up to 20% of complete hydatidiform mole pregnancies. About 15% of chorioadenoma destruens cases metastasize and require chemotherapy. Signs and symptoms of invasive hydatidiform mole include heavy or prolonged postpartum bleeding and increasing serum beta HCG levels in the postpartum period. Sonography is helpful to evaluate the location and extent of uterine wall invasion by molar tissue.

Anembryonic Pregnancy

An anembryonic pregnancy (referenced in the past as a blighted ovum) suggests an early failed pregnancy. In this situation, the embryo failed to grow, or death occurred before it could even be seen with ultrasound technology. In either case, the ultrasound will exhibit a gestational sac without a yolk sac or embryo. An embryo with cardiac activity should be seen during a transvaginal exam when the mean sac diameter (MSD) is greater than 16 mm. A yolk sac should be visible when the MSD is 8 mm or greater when using the same technique. Transabdominally, an embryo with positive fetal heart tones should be visualized when the MSD is 25 mm or greater. If an empty gestational sac is visualized and the measurements are less than the aforementioned parameters, then a follow-up ultrasound should be performed, and serial beta human chorionic gonadotropin levels should be measured. These serial exams will help clinicians determine if the empty gestational sac is due to an extremely early intrauterine pregnancy or an ectopic pregnancy with an associated false gestational sac.

Abnormal Gestation Sac

Early pregnancy abnormalities or complications may first be suspected when a gravid female complains of vaginal bleeding, pain or fever. This usually prompts evaluation with sonography. Gestational sacs that are anywhere other than the intrauterine position, are abnormal. If gestational sac size or visualization does not correlate with beta-hCG levels, consider an abnormality. If a gestational sac is at least 8 mm with no yolk sac or at least 16 mm without sonographic visualization of an embryo, the pregnancy is not developing normally. Furthermore, if a 5 mm or greater embryo is visualized but without cardiac activity, this is abnormal. Many of the above findings warrant correlation with beta-hCG and repeat sonography evaluation in a few days to support and confirm diagnosis. The exception to repeat sonography would be extrauterine implantation and ectopic pregnancy findings, which would warrant immediate action.

Ultrasound Indicators of Abnormal Yolk Sac

An early intrauterine pregnancy will be demonstrated on an ultrasound exam as an anechoic sac that correlates with the gestational sac. The next structure that will be identified within the gestational sac with ultrasound is the yolk sac. During an endovaginal ultrasound, the yolk sac is visualized during the fifth week. The ultrasound operator should examine not only the size of the yolk sac, but also how it is displayed sonographically. Yolk sacs that have an unusually large diameter (greater than 6 mm) may be associated with fetal demise. Yolk sacs should not be calcified, echogenic (except for the rim), asymmetrical, or absent if the mean sac diameter exceeds 8 mm. If any abnormality of a yolk sac is demonstrated, serial ultrasound exams should be performed because a full-term pregnancy could still be possible.

Subchorionic Hemorrhage

Subchorionic hemorrhage in early pregnancy is an abnormal sonographic finding. A subchorionic hemorrhage is basically blood or a blood clot found collected between the uterine wall and the outside of the chorionic membrane. This blood may then leak through the cervical canal, thus causing the gravid female to complain of vaginal bleeding and often prompting an ultrasound. In the embryonic stage, a subchorionic hemorrhage is the most common sonographic finding. Prognosis depends on three factors: clot size, gestational age, and maternal age. Miscarriage is more likely the larger the subchorionic hemorrhage, the older the mom, and the later the finding (late first trimester, early second trimester).

Intrauterine Contraceptive Device (IUCD) with Pregnancy

Although the purpose of an IUCD is to prevent pregnancy, sonographers should be aware of the possibility of a pregnancy occurring with an IUCD in place. If this happens, it is important to evaluate for an ectopic pregnancy because this is one risk of having an IUCD. If an intrauterine pregnancy is noted on the transvaginal ultrasound, the operator should check for a viable pregnancy and determine the age of gestation. The sonographer should also document the position of the IUCD. It is important to check for a bicornuate uterus because, in rare instances, it is possible to have a correctly positioned IUCD in one horn of the uterus with a pregnancy in the other in cases in which the patient and physician were not aware of this anatomical anomaly.

Incomplete or Missed Abortion

If a physician suspects retained products of conception (RPOC), an ultrasound will be ordered. Although the uterus will be measured during this exam, uterine size is not an indicator of RPOC because the size of the uterus will vary after childbirth. Sonographers should carefully evaluate the endometrial canal for placental tissue that may have a hyperechoic appearance. The endometrium will be thickened (8–13 mm) in positive cases of RPOC. A thickened endometrium or endometrial mass should also be evaluated with color or power Doppler because an increase in vascularity is a great indicator of RPOC. Other findings of RPOC are a complex mass, which could be from the placenta, necrotic tissue, or blood that has clotted and remains in the endometrium. There is a low probability of an incomplete abortion if a patient is not bleeding or if hyperechoic material is not visualized within the endometrium.

A missed abortion (embryonic demise) is used to describe a pregnancy that is no longer progressing as expected. An ultrasound will be ordered when there is an absence of fetal heart tones or if a patient is measuring smaller than expected during a clinical exam. Patients may or may not be experiencing vaginal bleeding at the time. A transvaginal ultrasound is the preferred method to determine a viable pregnancy in the first trimester. If an embryo is visualized and the crown rump length is greater than 4 mm, cardiac activity should be observed. If the crown rump length measures more than 4 mm, but a heartbeat is not visualized on ultrasound, it is assumed to be a nonviable pregnancy. It is suggested to have a physician or other operator observe in these situations. If no personnel are available, a video clip should be recorded. If a gestational sac is present, the yolk sac should be evident when the mean sac diameter reaches 8 mm. If the mean sac diameter measures greater than 16 mm, fetal heart tones should be present. If an embryo never develops, it is called a blighted ovum.

Chromosomal Anomalies

Trisomy 18 and 13

Trisomy 18, also termed Edward's syndrome, with an incidence of 1 in every 3,000 births. It is 3 times more common in females and holds a poor prognosis, with 90% not surviving beyond the first year of life. Sonographic evidence of trisomy 18 includes: multiple congenital heart and kidney defects, abnormally small placenta, excess amniotic fluid, low-set ears, clenched hands, micrognathia, and microcephaly. Trisomy 13, also called Patau syndrome, is another congenital and chromosomal defect with a poor prognosis. An estimated 80% of trisomy 13 babies do not survive beyond the first month of life. Incidence is about 1 in 5,000 births. Sonographic characteristics of trisomy 13 include: multiple cardiac defects, single umbilical artery, holoprosencephaly, cleft lip and palate, multiple eye and ear defects, polydactyly, and situs inversus.

Trisomy 21

Trisomy 21, perhaps more commonly termed Down syndrome is the most common chromosomal and congenital syndrome. Estimated incidence is 1 in every 730 births. The incidence rises dramatically to 1 in 75 pregnancies with a maternal age greater than 40 years. A large number of cases are diagnosed at birth, as fetal sonographic findings are vague and sometimes nonspecific. The best chance for prenatal diagnosis is amniocentesis, AFP, and triple screen tests. If the aforementioned tests are positive, a number of sonographic findings may support the diagnosis of Down syndrome. The following sonographic findings may be associated with trisomy 21: shorter-than-expected-for gestational age femur and humerus, underdeveloped 5th middle phalanx, dilated renal pelvis, thick nuchal fold, disproportionate short head, echogenic bowel and left intraventricular region, underdeveloped nasal bones, absent duodenal opening, and multiple heart defects.

Underdeveloped digits, specifically the 5th finger, may be a sonographic finding in the diagnosis of Down syndrome. When sonographically evaluating this, measurements of the middle 4th phalanx and the middle 5th phalanx should be taken. If the measurement of the 5th middle phalanx is only about 60% of that of the 4th middle phalanx, suspect Down syndrome. Brachycephaly is a common finding in Down syndrome; however, clear-cut definitions and measurements of the cephalic index have not been determined. The most common sonographic cardiac findings in Down syndrome are: atrioventricular canal defects and an echogenic portion in the left ventricle in the area of the papillary muscle.

There has been some correlation between sonographic findings of an increased angle between iliac bones and Down syndrome. However, this is a difficult measurement due to varying iliac angles that are dependent on varied sonographic planes. Sonographic plane and measurement parameters have not been established. Up to 70% of Down syndrome fetuses have been observed to have an underdeveloped nasal bridge. Proposed calculations based on nasal bone length and biparietal diameter have limitations with test specificity, sensitivity, and false-positive rates. a sonographic finding of duodenal atresia suggests a 30% risk of the fetus having Down syndrome. This finding is not available until at least the 22nd gestational week and therefore is not useful for pregnancy continuation or termination planning but may be used in conjunction with other findings to ready and educate the parents on having a child with Down syndrome.

Sonographic Scoring

A scoring system has been formulated based on the presence of a number of sonographic findings and their correlation with chromosomal disorders, with a slightly higher specificity for trisomy 21. The scoring system takes into account the presence of 7 sonographic findings: cardiac or duodenal defect, thickened nuchal fold, decreased femur length, dilated renal pelvis, choroid plexus cyst, and echogenic bowel. Each of these is given a score of one or two. If a fetus scores a > 2, amniocentesis is recommended. The higher the score is the greater the likelihood for Down syndrome. Although many other chromosomal anomalies would score high using this method, it is likely that these other disorders would be accompanied by more extreme organ and structural defects.

Independent sonographic findings have been rated on their correlation-to and likelihood ratio for developing Down syndrome. These likelihood ratios are not based on "grouped" findings or their correlation with amniocentesis results, AFP testing, and triple screen results. If one of the sonographic findings is not present, the risk of the fetus developing Down syndrome increases by 50% or 40% of its pre-sonographic marker. The isolated sonographic finding of nuchal thickening increases the odd of a fetus having Down syndrome by a factor of 11. Other independent ratios include: echogenic bowel increases likelihood by 6.7, decreased humeral length increases ratio by 5.1, decreased femoral length by 1.5, intracardiac echogenicity with a 1.8 ratio, and dilated renal pelvis has a likelihood ratio of 1.5.

X-Linked Diseases

An X-linked recessive disorder, since it is contained on the X-chromosome only, will be seen in more males than females. If a mother carries one abnormal X-chromosome and the father does not have the disorder, the male child has a 50% chance of displaying the disorder and a female child of the same parents has a 50% chance of carrying the disorder. An X-linked dominant disorder is more likely seen in females. A male with an X-linked dominant disorder will pass the disease on to all of his daughters and none of his sons, regardless of the mother's status. A mother with an X-linked disorder, assuming an unaffected father, gives both a male fetus and a female fetus a 50% chance of displaying the disease.

Autosomal Disorders

An autosomal recessive disorder is caused when each parent contributes an abnormal gene to one of the non-sex chromosomes of the child. In this case, the child will display the disorder. If only one parent contributes the abnormal gene to the chromosomal pair, the child will be a carrier of the defective gene but will not display symptoms of the disorder. If both parents carry the abnormal gene, the child has a 25% chance of displaying the disorder. An autosomal dominant disorder is present in a child when he or she receives a defective gene from one parent. Usually that parent also displays the disorder, since it is dominant. If one parent does not carry the defective gene, and the other parent has the chromosomal disorder (one defective gene and one normal gene), the child has a 50% chance of displaying the autosomal dominant disorder.

Jeune and Ellis-Van Creveld Syndromes

Jeune syndrome is an autosomal recessive disorder occurring in 1 in every 100,000 births. It has a poor prognosis, usually secondary to respiratory and renal problems. It is marked by many of the characteristics of skeletal dysplasia with markedly short and horizontally placed ribs, giving the thorax a cloverleaf appearance on fetal ultrasound. Ellis-Van Creveld syndrome is a rare autosomal recessive skeletal dysplasia marked by sonographic findings of shortened distal limbs and polydactyly of the feet. There is an increased incidence in the Amish and prognosis depends on degree of associated defects of the heart and lungs. Postnatally, one will observe characteristic anomalies of the hairline, teeth spacing and nails.

Meckel-Gruber Syndrome and Triploidy

Meckel-Gruber syndrome is a rare genetic disorder linked to chromosome 17 abnormalities. Worldwide incidence has huge variability with the highest incidence (1 in 9,000) seen in the Finnish population. The multiple defects associated with Meckel-Gruber syndrome are not compatible with life. Common sonographic findings include: polycystic kidneys, occipital encephalocele, postaxial polydactyly, genital abnormalities, cleft lip and palate, multiple central nervous system defects, and a fibrotic liver. Triploidy is a lethal fetal diagnosis occurring in about 1% of all pregnancies. A large percentage of triploidy cases result in a miscarriage or termination. Sonographic findings in triploidy will always reveal severe intrauterine growth restriction and some degree of molar gestation. Sonographic defects in all major organ systems are likely.

Turner Syndrome

Turner syndrome is a genetic disorder seen in females only. It may also be termed XO syndrome, Monosomy X, and gonadal dysgenesis. The incidence is 1 in 2,000 live births. There is a high rate of miscarriage in fetuses with Turner syndrome, miscarriage and prognosis is highly dependent on the presence and degree of fetal hydrops and pleural effusion. A potential sonographic finding associated with XO syndrome is cystic hygroma, which refers to multiple serous fluid collections, particularly around the shoulders and neck. Heart and kidney defects are probable sonographic findings in Turner syndrome.

Review Video: Turner Syndrome
Visit mometrix.com/academy and enter code: 802369

Obstetrics - Second/Third Trimester

Normal Anatomy and Physiology

Antepartum Ultrasound Examination

The AIUM guidelines for equipment and documentation for antepartum sonographic evaluation are much like those of any ultrasound evaluation. They include use of real-time equipment and use of appropriate transducer, using the lowest exposure required to gain the most accurate information. Testing should be done only in situations that are medically necessary or as per protocol screening guidelines. Appropriate infectious disease control and sterile measures must be followed. Detailed documentation of all findings, measurements and tests should accompany the patient's medical record. All images should be clearly labeled with the minimum patient identifiers (name and date of birth), exam date and image details.

Imaging Barriers

Advanced technology and techniques have made accurate sonographic images a reality over the past several decades. However, even technology has not quite overcome maternal obesity. Furthermore, fetal movement and position cannot be controlled for, thus limiting visualization of certain anatomy. Sonographic image quality may be compromised depending on the amount of amniotic fluid. Optimal sonography requires the operator to first assess fetal positioning. From there, the best plane and axis by which to view a particular fetal anatomy may be established. Use of real-time equipment is optimal as well as appropriate transducers and parameters.

Second and Third Trimester

AIUM guidelines for ultrasound in the second and third trimester include real-time imaging with evaluation and documentation of fetal number, position, amniotic fluid measurements and fetal activity (including heart rate). If sonographic gestational age has not already been determined in the first trimester, second trimester measurements are the last chance for the most accurate findings. Gestational age can be determined with head circumference and/or femur measurements. Fetal weight estimates can be determined by measurements of abdominal circumference. Do not overlook the importance of routine examination and documentation of cervix and adnexal structures. If readily visualized, include any other organ findings and measurements including brain and heart details.

Gestational Dating

Sonographic gestational age determination in the second or third trimester is most accurate with biparietal diameter measurements. Measurements of fetal head circumference and femur length may be supportive to the biparietal diameter measurements. Measurements from poor or suboptimal images should not be included. If the fetal age estimate is already known, it should not come into play when obtaining sonographic images and measurements. This recommendation arises from the tendency of a sonographer to alter measurement technique, repeat measurements, and second guess good measurements if they do not fit with the known gestational age. It is recommended that the sonographer remain unbiased to gestational age.

Placenta and Umbilical Cord

Role of Placenta

The placenta is the fetal lifeline. It allows for fetal survival, growth, development, nutrition, oxygen and carbon dioxide exchange, waste removal, hormone production, and protection from toxins and infections. This is all done through the placental connection to the uterus and umbilical cord, these allow for connection to the mother's blood supply. Due to the dependent nature of the fetal survival on the health of the placenta, routine monitoring with ultrasound is necessary. With sonographic exam of the placental, a number of points should be noted, including: placental size, shape, weight, position, and attachments.

Placental Size and Appearance

The normal placenta is flat and circular and weighs approximately one pound. The thickness in millimeters usually correlates with the gestational age in weeks; therefore, the placenta should not exceed 40 mm thickness. Suboptimal viewing planes, contractions, and increased or decreased amounts of amniotic fluid may hamper accurate placental thickness measurements. Abnormal placental thickness may be seen in diabetes, hemorrhage, infection, maternal anemia, incompatible blood groups, and chromosomal abnormalities. Decreased amniotic fluid and contraction may make the placenta appear falsely thickened. Decreased placental thickness may indicate hypertension, diabetes, toxemia or infection, chromosomal abnormalities, and growth restrictions. Increased amniotic fluid may give the placenta a falsely thin appearance.

Umbilical Cord

Anatomically, the umbilical cord is comprised of two arteries that transport deoxygenated blood from fetus to placenta. The umbilical cord also contains one vein that transports oxygen-rich blood from the placenta to the maternal liver. Wharton's jelly surrounds these vessels within the umbilical cord, acting as a connective tissue and protectant. Sonographically, the umbilical cord can be viewed as early as 8 weeks. It will about the same length as the crown-rump length and appears thick and straight, maintaining a diameter of less than 2 cm throughout pregnancy. Thorough sonographic evaluation of the umbilical cord is important in identifying a number of possible fetal abnormalities and pregnancy complications.

Amniotic Fluid

Amniotic fluid surrounds a fetus throughout pregnancy and is constantly recirculated by the fetus "inhaling" and swallowing it and returning it by "exhalation" and urination. The amount of amniotic fluid increases to a peak volume of 800 mL at 34 weeks gestation then decreases slightly. By delivery, about 600 mL still remains, surrounding the fetus. Amniotic fluid functions to protect and cushion the fetus from outside trauma. Amniotic fluid also maintains a consistent temperature for the fetus, to prevent against heat loss. Fetal movement is made possible by the amniotic fluid, which allows for fetal musculoskeletal development. Amniotic fluid is also largely responsible for fetal lung development.

Several methods exist for the estimation of amniotic fluid volume. Amniotic fluid volume estimation is primarily attempted through sonographic routes and many methods are qualitative in nature, which limits their use and consistency. If a qualitative method is being used, the subjective findings are ranked on a scale of 1 to 5. One represents no amniotic fluid and five represent severe excess of amniotic fluid. The AFI (amniotic fluid index) attempts to quantify the amount of amniotic fluid. The AFI is determined by adding the depth of the largest vertical pockets from four areas of the uterus. An AFI of < 5 cm indicates insufficient amniotic fluid and > 20 cm indicates excessive amniotic fluid.

Determining Fetal Lie

Fetal lie is the comparison of the long axis of the fetus to the maternal long axis with the most common being a longitudinal lie. Fetal lie must be determined while performing an OB ultrasound so that the sonographer can ascertain the normal anatomy. Fetal lie is not a parameter that can be controlled by the sonographer (nor can the amount of amniotic fluid or maternal body habitus), which all may limit an exam. Some anatomical structures are more readily visualized with the fetus in a certain position. Starting in a longitudinal scan at the cervix, determine the general position of the fetus (breech, cephalic, transverse, or oblique). Next, determine the position of the spine. If the fetus is in a transverse or oblique orientation, then manipulation of the transducer will be necessary to find the long axis. During first- and second-trimester exams, the fetus will often move, so it is important to be aware of the body plane when trying to find the best window for an anatomical survey.

Importance of Establishing Fetal Presentation

Fetal presentation is the body part of the fetus that is leading into the birth canal. Fetal lie and presentation are often established at the beginning of an OB exam so that the sonographer can determine if the anatomical structures are in the correct places. The most common fetal lie and presentation are longitudinal and cephalic. This indicates that the long axis of the fetus is parallel to the long axis of the mother with the head closest to the cervix. A fetus that is breech is also parallel to the long axis of the mother, but, instead, the buttocks (frank breech) or at least one of the feet (footling breech) are the body parts that are closest to the cervix. In cases of a transverse lie, the fetal shoulder, arm, or back could be the presenting part. There is a greater risk of mortality with breech presentations, so it is important to provide this information to the doctors because they may opt to turn the fetus prior to birth or may perform a cesarean section.

Head and Face

Intracranial Structures

Septum pellucidum is a thin membranous structure, triangular in shape and vertical in position, which separates the brains lateral ventricles.

Corpus callosum is a white matter structure that connects the left and right cerebral hemispheres of the brain.

Cisterna magna, also called the cerebellomedullary cistern, is an opening in the subarachnoid space that results in a cavity between the brains cerebellum and medulla.

Cerebral peduncle is a term used to describe the tegmentum, crus cerebri, substantia nigra, and the pretectum. In other words, it is all midbrain structures except the tectum.

Cerebellum is the posterior portion of the brain comprised of two lateral hemispheres connected by the vermis.

Imaging Fetal Head and Face

Sonographic evaluation of the fetal facial features is becoming increasingly routine, especially if other fetal anomalies are suspected. For optimal sonographic viewing and facial descriptions, it is necessary to view the fetal face and head in multiple planes. Some fetal features are viewed more optimally through these planes. For example, the axial view probably provides the most detailed examination of the most superficial features: forehead, orbits, nose, cheek and jaw bones, lips and tongue, and neck. The mid and hard palate, tongue, mandible, neck soft-tissue structures, and more detailed view of the lips and nose can be obtained from the frontal plane. Three-dimensional imaging allows for a better profile view of the fetal head and face, and often allow for better imaging of the ears and neck structures.

Fetal Cranium

The fetal head and brain are a commonly imaged entity due to gestational age determination imaging of the biparietal diameter and head circumference. Taking these measurements further, the sonographer evaluates the rest of the cranial contents from superior to inferior. The falx and tentorium are dural structures that should be noted, and are necessary landmarks for biparietal measurements anyway. These are usually best viewed in the axial plane. Transaxial views allow for optimal imaging of the ventricles. The atrial measurements remain relatively consistent throughout the second and third trimesters. The temporal and occipital horns of the lateral ventricles are readily viewed.

Fetal Cerebellum and Ears

Sonographic viewing of the cerebellum during the second and third trimesters is best accomplished in the transverse plane. In this view, fluid is a normal finding between the hemispheres of the cerebellum and the occipital bone of the fetal skull. The sonographer will already be in this area when evaluating the nuchal translucency measurements. The transverse plane images the cerebellum with the cavum septum pellucidum anterior. The cavum septum pellucidum lies midline between the lateral ventricles, if filled with fluid, and is not evident at term. External ear structures can be sonographically imaged in great detail. Care must be taken to thoroughly describe the plane in which the ear image is being obtained as well as identifying adjacent landmarks, so as not to misdiagnose a normal fetal ear as an encephalocele.

Brain and Cranium Development

Although the fetal nervous system development starts very early, the earliest sonographic evidence of this is at the 5th week of gestation. At this time, the fetal spine can be visualized and the neural tube is forming within this. At about 13 weeks, the brain ventricles can be visualized at about their maximal transverse diameter of about 7 mm. The rest of the fetal brain grows and develops progressively around the ventricles throughout the pregnancy. The choroid plexus will continue its growth from the anterior position moving posteriorly as gestation progresses, eventually dominating the posterior ventricular region. At about the time the ventricles can be viewed, the corpus callosum begins its development. Furthermore, sonography at 10-15 weeks should visualize the fetal calvarium. These developments can all be monitored as the corpus callosum continues to develop through the 20th gestational week. At this stage (18-20 weeks) the cavi septi pellucidi can be seen beneath the corpus callosum. The inferior cerebellar vermis can also be seen at the 18th week.

Diencephalons and Rhombencephalon

Diencephalon refers to the midline portion of the human brain, superior to the brainstem. The diencephalon contains the forebrain structures such as the hypothalamus, thalamus, subthalamus, epithalamus, pretectum, and a portion of the pituitary gland. The diencephalon is responsible for much of the autonomic and visceral functions in the human body. The rhombencephalon is also known as the hindbrain. The rhombencephalon is comprised of the cerebellum, pons, and medulla oblongata. These structures contain many of the cranial nerves. It is often further broken down into the metencephalon and myelencephalon. The rhombencephalon is responsible for: complex muscle movements, simple learning, autonomic function, attention, and sleep.

Prosencephalon and Mesencephalon

The prosencephalon is also known as the forebrain and is therefore the most anterior located portion of the brain. When it divides, during embryonic development, it forms the diencephalons and the telencephalon. When the prosencephalon fails to divide in the developing fetus, holoprosencephaly (often times with facial anomalies) occurs. The prosencephalon is responsible for directing impulses to our senses, personality, and intelligence. The mesencephalon is also known as the midbrain and made of the tectum and tegmentum. The mesencephalon helps process visual and auditory cues.

Sonographic Facial Features

Accurate imaging of facial features, particularly the nose and lips, is important medically for the diagnosis of cleft lip deformities. These deformities can be best viewed in the coronal plane, along with the maxilla, anterior jawbone and the orbits. Many fetal facial structures can be identified even when positioning is not optimal. Optimal viewing of facial bones, nasal bones, jawbone, and soft tissue of the face are obtained with a fetal profile angle. Imaging the fetal face in the axial plane allows for optimal images of the anterior palate, oropharynx, tongue, and the same structures viewed in the coronal plane. The ears, eyebrows, eyelids and cheeks are often viewed with good clarity. By about 20 weeks, tooth buds along the gingival ridge can be seen. By the late second trimester and early third trimester it is not unusual to view intraorbital contents with great clarity.

Development of Fetal Face

Facial structures develop in the fetus as early as 6 weeks gestation. At this stage the orbits are seen on the sides of the face. The nasal and palate structures also start out high and on the sides of the face at this stage. It is at about this time that a cleft palate may develop if these structures do not migrate normally to their midline position. As early as gestational week 8, the above aforementioned structures will turn to bone, and by about the 11th gestational week, sonographic examination of these structures becomes feasible. Of particular sonographic interest at this stage is an orbital measurement. Maximal orbital diameter should be about equal and the distance between the orbits should be about that of the orbital diameter itself.

Choroid Plexus Cysts

Choroid plexus cysts describe fluid-filled sacs that develop in the choroid glomi, the portion of the brain that makes cerebrospinal fluid. The choroid glomi can be seen on ultrasound as early as five weeks gestation. The fetal brain essentially forms around these structures. Small choroid plexus cysts, in and of themselves, are generally not an ominous finding and they always resolve through the pregnancy. However, if the choroid plexus cysts are large enough to be seen on ultrasound, they are thought to be associated with an increased risk of fetal chromosomal disorders.

Fetal Intracranial Tumors

The most common fetal intracranial tumor is a teratoma, although all fetal intracranial tumors are extremely rare. Fetal intracranial tumor should be suspected anytime sonography detects hydrocephalus or any mass-occupying lesion. Intracranial tumors may have low echogenicity on ultrasound. Prognosis is poor for all types of fetal intracranial tumors. In utero intracranial hemorrhage is also extremely rare and is usually the result of maternal problems. Fetal intracranial calcifications are a rare, late pregnancy sonographic finding. Intracranial calcifications are usually secondary to infectious agents. Associated sonographic findings may include lateral ventricular enlargement and a small-for-gestational-age head.

Vein of Galen Aneurysm

A vein of Galen aneurysm in the fetal brain is not an aneurysm at all; rather it is a vascular malformation. This arteriovenous malformation shunts blood into the dilated vein of Galen from the cerebral arteries. The malformation develops by the 11th gestational week, but is not likely to be detected before the 32nd gestational week and more often until after birth. The best chance for fetal detection is with Doppler ultrasound. In the delivered infant, often the first sign of vein of Galen aneurysm is congestive heart failure. Although rare in terms of overall vascular malformations, vein of Galen aneurysm accounts for up to 30% of all fetal and infant vascular malformations.

Structures Assessed in the Fetal Neck

The 3D and 4D ultrasounds have greatly improved the visualization of structures in the neck that can be assessed during an OB ultrasound. Gray-scale imaging in two planes is still very useful to determine any abnormalities of the shape of the neck. The first thing a sonographer may want to examine is the contour of the neck. Any interruption of the normal contour of the neck region may be the first clue of an abnormality. Next, it is important for the ultrasound technologist to inspect for any mass (cystic or solid) that is projecting from the neck. Normal anatomical structures that can be assessed in the neck region of a fetus include the esophagus, trachea, thyroid, carotid arteries, and lymphatic sacs of the jugular region. The nuchal fold can be measured in the posterior neck, and the cervical vertebrae are visualized as well.

Measurements of the Orbits

During an evaluation of the fetal face, the sonographer must also look at the orbits. Typically, an evaluation of the orbits does not require any measurements, unless the ultrasound operator believes that the orbits are too close together (hypotelorism), too far apart (hypertelorism), or appear smaller than expected (microphthalmia). Evaluating the orbits is subjective, but a good rule of thumb to follow is that the bony orbits should be the same size and the space between the two orbits should be the same width as one orbit. If the width between the orbits is concerning to the sonographer, then it is possible to provide measurements because they can be compared to standardized recorded normal values. Sonographers should be aware that holoprosencephaly may be present when hypotelorism is suspected. In exams that suggest hypertelorism, the sonographer should look for a number of chromosomal malformations or median cleft face syndrome.

The orbits are not routinely measured during an OB ultrasound, but in certain cases these measurements may provide insight on various fetal abnormalities. During ultrasounds performed later in the pregnancy, the internal structures of the orbits may be identified, such as the lens and optic nerve. If a fetus is diagnosed with hypertelorism (a greater amount of space separating the orbits), the sonographer should interrogate further to rule out median cleft face syndrome. If hypotelorism is present, the space between the eyes is reduced. Orbital measurements can be taken at a level that runs parallel (but below) the biparietal diameter and head circumference in a transverse axial cut. There should be two orbits that are symmetrical in size with the space between them being about the diameter of an orbit. The inner orbital measurement is taken from the inside of an eye socket to the inside of the contralateral eye socket (also known as the interocular distance). The outer orbital diameter is measured at the outside edges of each eye socket; it is also referred to as the binocular distance. These measurements vary with gestational age, so it is important to have a good reference for comparison.

Measuring the Nasal Bone

The nasal bone should be documented on an OB ultrasound because fetuses are at a higher risk for having trisomy 18 or 21 when they have an absent or hypoplastic (shortened) nasal bone. This absence or shortening of the nasal bone is apparent in more than half of the cases of fetuses with trisomy 18 or 21, but there is a higher association with trisomy 21. While imaging the fetal face, the nasal bone can be identified as parallel reflectors best visualized on a midsagittal plane. In the second trimester, the length of the nasal bone increases with increasing gestational age, but some ethnicities tend to demonstrate a shortened nasal bone in the absence of chromosomal anomalies. Both 2D and 3D ultrasound can be used to provide the best images of the nasal bone. Skeletal dysplasia may demonstrate a nose that appears to be flat as well as the appearance of micrognathia and a forward-protruding forehead.

Heart

Embryonic Cardiac Activity

Cardiac activity correlates highly with embryo/fetal well-being. This correlation exists because it is a marker of adequate fetal oxygenation. In the early embryonic stage, transvaginal sonograph may be the best way to determine cardiac rate. In the fetal stage, better methods of fetal heart monitoring exist. In the first 6 gestational weeks, embryonic heart rate is at its lowest at 100 – 120 beats per minute. The normal embryonic heart rate peaks to about 140 beats per minute between gestational weeks 8 and 10. If embryonic cardiac rate remains less than 100 bpm in the first 6 weeks; the rate of miscarriage increases. Likewise, miscarriage is more likely with cardiac rates less than 120 bpm between 6 and 8 weeks gestation.

Review Video: Fetal Heart Rate
Visit mometrix.com/academy and enter code: 980576

Fetal Vessels and Esophagus

Optimal viewing of the great vessels in a fetus can be obtained after imaging the four-chamber view of the fetal heart. From the fetal heart images, the transducer should be moved toward the fetal head. This places the transducer in a transverse axial plane. From here, images of the ascending and descending thoracic aorta, the pulmonary artery, the superior vena cava, and the ductus arteriosus can be obtained. The branching vessels from the aortic arch can be imaged best from the sagittal view. From the descending thoracic aorta, moving the transducer anterior from this landmark can sometimes allow for visualization of portions of the esophagus. However, the esophagus is much more difficult to view than the great vessels of the fetus.

Evaluating the Fetal Heart

On routine fetal sonography, the heart should be evaluated in as much detail as the fetal positioning will allow. At minimum, a cross-sectional four-chamber view should be obtained. Chambers should be symmetrical, valves should be documented, and oftentimes the foramen ovale may be seen. A short-axis view through the sagittal plane (with rotation and depending on the level) allows for more detailed evaluation of the left ventricle, ventricular septum, aortic arch, and the mitral valve. Viewing of the outflow tracts is difficult with routine screening, and may be better obtained with off-axis views, segmental views, and/or Doppler studies.

With routine fetal heart sonography the fetal heart should consume one-third of the thorax in the cross-sectional plane. The atria should be of about equal size and appearance. The ventricles should be of equal size. The foramen ovale should be slightly bowed towards the left atria. The internal left ventricle is smooth and the right internal ventricle is rough appearing. Two papillary muscles should be visualized within the left ventricle. The outflow tracts will demonstrate the crossing of the great arteries. Furthermore, the pulmonary artery should show division into its right and left branches.

Thorax and Abdomen

Fetal Larynx, Trachea, Diaphragm and Lungs

The second and third trimester sonograph allows for visualization of the larynx. This is most readily viewed as the constricted portion of the fluid column of the trachea superiorly. The fluid-filled hypopharynx allows for easy viewing of the larynx. If visible, the trachea will be filled with fluid as well. It may be optimal to trace the distal trachea from its location behind the aortic arch, and image it moving superiorly. The fetal diaphragm separates the lungs from the liver and ultimately the chest from the abdominal contents. Check for diaphragmatic herniation. Although the lungs and liver may be seen on ultrasound from early in the second trimester, the later in pregnancy they are imaged, the more they separate out to define themselves with increasing echogenicity of the lungs.

Thoracic Development

The healthy fetal lung develops under the following conditions: sufficient thorax cavity, normal fetal breathing, fetal pulmonary fluid production, and normal amniotic fluid amounts. The first signs of fetal lung development occur as early as the 5th gestational week with the development of the lung buds. By the 20th week, all of the bronchi will have developed. The alveoli develop through the 24th week. However, it is not until the 35th gestational week that sufficient amounts of lung surfactant are present. Lung surfactant is crucial to the maintenance of breathing and air pressure. Sonographically, normal fetal lungs should be moderately homogeneous and more echogenic than the nearby liver. The lungs should occupy one third of the thoracic cavity with the right lung being slightly larger than the left lung, due to heart placement.

Assessing the Fetal Diaphragm

The diaphragm is a muscle that is a necessary component of the respiratory system that differentiates the thoracic cavity from the abdominal cavity. Sonographically, the diaphragm should present as a hypoechoic, uninterrupted line separating the fetal heart and lungs from the abdominal organs such as the liver and the stomach. Congenital diaphragmatic hernias (CDHs) are one abnormality that are ruled out when evaluating the fetal chest; these are the most prevalent anomaly of the diaphragm. Although they are more common on the left side, CDHs may develop on the right side or could even be bilateral in some cases. If present, a sonographer often sees the stomach bubble or loops of bowel in the chest. It is important to diagnose CDHs during an OB ultrasound because there is a high mortality rate due to the associated pulmonary hypertension and hypoplasia. The diaphragm is an important structure to watch during a biophysical profile because the sonographer must see an episode of breathing for at least 30 seconds within a 30-minute exam window.

Fetal Abdomen

Abdominal sonography is best performed in the transverse plane, and abdominal circumference is a common measurement. Fetal abdominal anatomy that may be visualized with ultrasound include: abdominal muscles, stomach, duodenum, colon, liver, umbilicus with cord insertion, kidneys and adrenal glands, ureters, bladder, abdominal aorta, and inferior vena cava. The muscular portion of the abdominal wall is hypoechoic and should not be confused with ascites. Fluid in the stomach, gallbladder and bladder are normal findings. Any other fluid-containing structure should be considered abnormal and further evaluated. The umbilical cord should contain three vessels identifiable via sonography.

Genitourinary System

Development of the kidneys of the fetal genitourinary system can be seen sonographically as early as 7 weeks gestation. By the 11th gestational week, the kidneys have located to their permanent anatomical location in the fetal flank, adjacent to the thoracolumbar spine. By 17 weeks gestation, the fetal kidneys are responsible for almost 100% of amniotic fluid production via fetal urination. Fetal urination and complete bladder emptying occurs at least twice per hour. Normal fetal kidney circumference remains slightly less than 1/3 of the fetal abdominal circumference measurements throughout pregnancy. Sonographically, the fetal kidneys should be readily imaged by the 14th week as individual, hypoechoic, elliptical structures. Many fetal kidney anomalies may not be apparent via sonographic evaluation until the third trimester.

Gastrointestinal System

During embryologic development, the GI (gastrointestinal) tract is discussed in three categories: foregut, midgut, and hindgut. The foregut comprises the most superior abdominal structures such as the esophagus, stomach, anterior duodenum, pancreas and liver. The midgut forms the rest of the duodenum, small intestine, and the first portion of the colon. The hindgut will give rise to the more inferior abdominal cavity structures including the colon, rectum, and portions of the genitourinary tract. the 6th gestational week sees foregut dilation. By the 12th gestational week, the midgut herniates into the umbilical cord at its base, rotates, and descends back into the abdominal cavity by the 14th gestational week.

Gastrointestinal Tract and Stomach

The fetal gastrointestinal system can be seen sonographically by the 14th gestational week. However, at this stage there is poor differentiation between large and small bowel, as it all appears echogenic. At 20 weeks gestation, the colon diameter measures up to 5 mm and steadily increases to about 18 mm by delivery. Sonographic differentiation is possible after 22 weeks by observing the meconium-filled colon. Normal sonographic position of the fetal stomach or foregut should be in the left upper quadrant, its position in relation to the heart apex (left side) is important to note.

The fetal stomach should be easily viewed via sonography after 14 gestational weeks. In the event of sonographic absence of the stomach, interval reevaluation should be scheduled and fetal anomalies considered. Anomalies that may be responsible for nonvisualization of the fetal stomach are largely centered on any condition that would impair fetal swallowing, central nervous system anomalies, and musculoskeletal defects. Other conditions that may not allow for sonographic visualization of the fetal stomach are: stomach displacement into chest or base of umbilical cord, an abnormally small stomach, reduced esophageal patency, decreased amniotic fluid production or failure to reach the amniotic cavity, and the presence of a normal stomach that has just emptied.

Fetal Liver, Gallbladder, Spleen, and Ascites

A sonographically normal appearing fetal liver should appear homogenous. Any hypoechoic areas signify an abnormal mass. Calcifications may be viewed as abnormal from vascular injury or infection. An enlarged fetal liver is abnormal and secondary to Rh disease, infection, and a number of syndromes. If the fetal gallbladder cannot be identified sonographically by 15 weeks, consider cystic fibrosis, or atresia somewhere in the surrounding GI tract. The normal fetal spleen is not always visualized sonographically; therefore, it is the presence of splenomegaly that would be an abnormal finding and suggest infection. The sonographic finding of fetal abdominal ascites is always an abnormal finding and can signify a number of conditions and therefore requires close evaluation of all other fetal structures.

Fetal Skeleton

The first sonographic signs of fetal bony development can be seen at 6 gestational weeks. Ossification of skeletal bone begins between gestational weeks 9 and 13, starting with the collarbone, skull, vertebrae, long bones, and pelvic girdle (usually in that order). Normally the change of fetal skeleton to bony material occurs earlier in the fetal female. Sonographic descriptors of abnormal fetal skeletal development may include: agenesis, duplication, abnormal differentiation, hypoplasia, hyperplasia, or constriction band presence. Furthermore, the individual descriptors above need to identify whether the abnormal skeletal condition affects a localized area or the entire fetal skeleton.

Fetal Spine

The fetal spine serves an important landmark for sonographic studies, as well as an important anatomical structure to evaluate and record to determine normal development. Determination of the continuity of the spinal column and the skin above it should be first determined in an overview in the transverse plane. Each vertebral body should be evaluated, along with the right and left posterior elements. These should be viewed in at least two different planes. by the second and third trimester, the spinal cord can be visualized under optimal sonographic conditions and fetal positioning. The spinal cord has bright margins and a central and is hypoechoic.

Fetal Pelvis

Sonography of the fetal pelvis includes the skeletal structures such as the iliac bones, pubic symphysis, and sacrum. The fetal pelvis also contains the urinary bladder, colon, rectum and pelvic vessels, which can be identified readily during the second and third trimester ultrasound. Imaging of the fetal pelvic vessels helps confirm the 3-vessel composition of the umbilical cord. The posterior fetal rectum and anterior fetal bladder are equally echogenic. If the fetal bladder is without fluid, it may be missed or confused with colonic and rectal structures.

Fetal Extremities

Sonographic evaluation of the extremities is important to monitor growth and screen for any abnormalities. The limbs (arms and legs) can usually be readily evaluated with ultrasound, and good images can be obtained in many planes. The hands, feet, fingers and toes must all be evaluated. Sonographs of the fetus may detect limb absence, abnormal number of digits, clubfoot, and fetal length. Normal fetal leg bones include a longer fibula distally. Proximally, the tibia and fibula are level. In the normal fetal forearm, a similar situation exists. The ulna is the longer bone. The ulna and radius are equal at the distal end, but the ulna extends beyond the radius proximally. Sonograms done later in the third trimester may show ossification centers; this is a sign of a mature fetus. Ossifications develop a few weeks earlier in the female fetus, and may be demonstrated as early as 32 weeks.

Evaluation of Fetal Hands and Fingers

Sonographic exams of the fetus will include a survey of both fetal hands. This should include the position of the thumb and fingers compared to the hands and wrists and the number of digits. Typically, the hands will demonstrate fingers that are slightly bent. The operator should try to capture images as the fetus opens and extends the fingers, and ideally it should be noted that the fetus opened the hand at least once during the exam. A fetus that does not open the hands completely during the course of the exam may be at a higher risk of trisomy 18. Also, any abnormalities concerning the fetal hands such as polydactyly (too many digits) should facilitate further investigation because they are often connected to aneuploidy. Whether abnormalities of the fingers (and toes) are an isolated incident or are an associated abnormality, parents can be better prepared for the situation once the baby is born.

Fetal Abnormalities

Multiple Gestations

Increased Complication Incidence

Multiple gestation pregnancies carry greater risk of low birth weight babies and preterm delivery. Approximately 60% of twins are delivered preterm. This percentage increases with increasing number of multiples. Most preterm multiples are considered 'low-birth-weight' which is less than 5 ½ pounds. Again, the higher the number of multiples and the earlier the preterm delivery, the lower the birth weight measurements. Even before birth, multiple gestations are at increased risk of complications. Monozygote twins are at increased risk for twin-to-twin-transfusion syndrome and birth defects. Other defects that may be seen in multiple gestations include: embolization syndrome, umbilical cord entanglement, vessel anastomoses, and acardiac parabiotic syndrome. Maternal risks such as preeclampsia and gestational diabetes also increase when carrying multiples versus singletons.

Twin Embolization Syndrome

Twin embolization syndrome (TES) is a condition that is most commonly associated with monozygote monochorionic twins. It is a condition in which one fetus dies, often secondary to twin-twin transfusion syndrome. The demise of the one fetus results in embolization placental fragments, fetal thromboplastin, and any other number of necrosed fetal fragments. This embolized matter affects the surviving fetus or twin in a number of ways. The more vascular organs of the living twin are most notably affected including the brain and kidneys. Twin embolization syndrome can result in a number of central nervous system defects and anomalies in the surviving fetus. Furthermore, anomalies throughout the GI system and abdominal cavity (especially necrotic in nature) and even limb defects occur in the remaining fetus when TES is present.

Acardiac Twin

The acardiac twin anomaly is also known as Twin-Reversed Arterial Perfusion sequence or TRAP sequence. TRAP sequence is seen in only about 1 in 35,000 births. It is seen in monozygotic monochorionic gestations. The TRAP sequence occurs when there is a venous and arterial anastomosis that results in retrograde deoxygenated blood flow to the acardiac twin. This results in significantly compromised development that is seen essentially in all major organ systems from the waist and up in the acardiac twin. These structural abnormalities are diagnostic on ultrasound as well as retrograde umbilical flow of the acardiac twin on Doppler studies. The other twin often develops normally.

Diagnosis of Acardiac Twinning with Ultrasound Imaging

Acardiac twinning is a complication that may only take place in a monozygotic twin pregnancy, and, of course, it will be of the same sex. Ultrasound indications of this malformation include the visualization of one twin that is extremely deformed, referred to as the acardiac twin. As the term acardiac suggests, this twin does not develop a heart, or the heart is severely malformed. Often, the superior body of this fetus has not been formed, and the head is either missing or microcephaly is present. The other twin is often fully developed and is referred to as the "pump" twin; this twin is at a higher risk for hydrops, polyhydramnios, or congestive heart failure. It is believed that this condition occurs as blood flows through an artery-to-artery anastomosis and a vein-to-vein anastomosis, and it is referred to as twin reversed arterial perfusion. The inferior portion of the acardiac twin tends to receive blood that is richer in oxygen, so these body parts are often well developed.

Cord Entanglement and Conjoined Twins

Umbilical cord entanglement syndrome is a condition seen in approximately 50% of monoamniotic twins. The risk is high in this situation because of the shared amniotic sac and thus the lack of membranous separation of the umbilical cords of the two fetuses. This results in twisting, tangling and even knotting of the two umbilical cords and resulting fetal complications and even mortality that would be associated with a compromised blood flow to and from the fetus(es). Conjoined twins are rare but may develop from the partial division of a single fertilized ovum. This rare condition is readily diagnosed with sonography. Sonography is important in determining twin attachment site and shared organs. Their anatomical conjunction site further classifies conjoined twins. Common attachment sites are the abdomen and thorax (omphalopagus and thoracopagus).

Common Abnormalities Associated with Multiple Gestations

Sonographers should understand that all multiple gestations are considered to be high-risk pregnancies not only for the fetuses, but also for the mother. Congenital abnormalities are found two to three times more often in pregnancies that are associated with twins than in a single gestation. Multiple gestations have escalated due to increasing maternal age and the use of infertility techniques. Like all obstetrical ultrasounds, it is important for the operator to determine the number of gestations as well as the presentation. It is also important to determine the number of amniotic sacs and placentas, which is more accurately identified in the first trimester. More anomalies are found in monozygotic pregnancies than those found in dizygotic pregnancies and include acardiac twinning, conjoined twins, twin-twin transfusion syndrome, vanishing twin, or a heterotopic multifetal pregnancy. It is important to correctly diagnose any anomaly as soon as possible so that the specialists can make the best decision for the patients.

Ultrasound Findings of Conjoined Twins

Conjoined twins are an unlikely occurrence in a monozygotic pregnancy that will only take place in the presence of one amnion and a single chorion. If a sonographer identifies a twin pregnancy but cannot see an amniotic membrane separating the fetuses in the presence of one placenta, this should be a consideration. Conjoined twins can never occur when the amniotic membrane is present or in the presence of more than one placenta. Ultrasound clues of conjoined twins include fetal heads that are aligned at the same height, bodies and organs that cannot be identified as separate entities, fetuses that demonstrate extension of the neck while facing their twin, demonstration of more than three vessels in one umbilical cord, and polyhydramnios. Conjoined twins are most often characterized as thoracopagus (the most frequent anomaly when fetuses are joined at the chest), thoraco-omphalopagus (joined at the chest and abdomen), omphalopagus (joined at the abdomen), and craniopagus (joined at the head).

Twin-Twin Transfusion Syndrome

Twin-twin transfusion syndrome (TTTS) may also be known as feto-fetal transfusion syndrome or twin oligohydramnios-polyhydramnios syndrome. TTTS is seen in monochorionic twins or higher multiples. TTTS is a condition in which one fetus receives a greater proportion of fetal nutrients and blood flow than the other, secondary to placental vessel anastomoses. This condition results in significant fetal morbidity and mortality for both fetuses. The donor fetus has complications associated with decreased blood flow and nutrition and is usually significantly smaller as a result of receiving its less-than-normal proportion of blood flow. The recipient twin is the larger fetus and experiences complications associated with increased volume because it receives a proportionately greater amount of blood flow than its twin. The main condition associated with increased volume is congestive heart failure (fetal or neonatal).

Ultrasound Findings of Twin-Twin Transfusion Syndrome

Twin-twin transfusion syndrome (TTTS) only takes place in monozygotic twins that share one placenta. This is a syndrome that actually affects the placenta instead of the twins, but because the blood flow is not dispersed evenly between the twins, it affects their growth differently. TTTS is believed to be caused when artery-to-vein anastomosis deflects blood flow away from one twin to the other. The connection tends to be from the umbilical arterial system of the twin that is displaying growth restriction, or the "donor" twin, to the larger "recipient's" umbilical vein. This shunting of blood creates a significant risk for both twins. Ultrasound findings will often reveal that a "donor" twin that is measuring smaller than expected is not moving and actually appears "stuck" in the presence of oligohydramnios. The larger "recipient" twin may have hydrops in the presence of polyhydramnios, with organomegaly and ascites.

Heterotopic Multifetal Pregnancy

A heterotopic multifetal pregnancy is a dangerous diagnosis in which an extrauterine pregnancy occurs simultaneously with an intrauterine pregnancy. This is a difficult clinical diagnosis, and like all ectopic pregnancies, if not correctly diagnosed it can be life-threatening. Transvaginal sonography is an important method to aid in this diagnosis. Sonographers must be aware of this phenomenon, especially with the prevalence of assisted reproductive methods that so many patients undergo. More cases of heterotopic multifetal pregnancies occur with those that have sought the assistance of fertility specialists or have had prior pelvic surgeries, but it may also take place in natural pregnancies. It is important that sonographers check for an ectopic pregnancy when an adnexal mass is seen or when free fluid is present. If the adnexal mass proves to be hyperemic and demonstrates a reduced resistive index, then a heterotopic pregnancy should be considered even when a normal intrauterine pregnancy has been identified.

Abnormal Amniotic Fluid Volume

Oligohydramnios indicates insufficient amounts of amniotic fluid, usually less than 300 mL. Oligohydramnios may be defined in a number of ways. If using the AFI, oligohydramnios is present if < 5 cm. If sonographic measurement of vertical pockets in the uterine quadrants are < 2 cm, consider oligohydramnios. Oligohydramnios may occur with abnormalities in fetal urinary tract and kidney development as well as intrauterine growth restriction. Polyhydramnios is the presence of excessive amounts of amniotic fluid, usually > 2000 mL. Using the AFI, polyhydramnios is defined as a measurement of > 20 cm. Polyhydramnios may occur in any situation in which the fetal ability to swallow and absorb amniotic fluid is compromised.

Abnormal Fetal Growth

Intrauterine Growth Restriction

Intrauterine growth restriction (IUGR) is a condition or term used to define a fetal weight that is below the 10th percentile for gestational age. This is determined by fetal weight and gestational age tables. Further definition of IUGR includes a fetal abdominal circumference measurement less than the 2.5 percentile. Intrauterine growth restriction should be differentiated from 'small-for-gestational-age'. If a fetus is small-for-gestational-age, they are otherwise healthy and have reached their appropriate growth potential. Usually a diagnosis of small-for-gestational-age is made retrospectively and after delivery and evaluation. IUGR carries a high risk for perinatal mortality and morbidity. Accurate and early diagnosis, however, can reduce mortality rates.

There are several risk factors for the development of intrauterine growth restriction. Anatomical/physiologic risk factors include a small maternal uterus and placental abnormalities. High altitude is considered an environmental risk. Poor maternal nutrition and/or maternal use of drugs, alcohol, tobacco products, and certain prescription medications increase the risk for development of IUGR. Furthermore, maternal vascular and heart disease, diabetes, kidney disease, asthma, GI disorders, and bleeding/clotting disorders can contribute to the development of IUGR. Previous miscarriage, multiple pregnancy, and maternal infections (viral, parasitic, and bacterial) are causative for IUGR. Complications during pregnancy such as preeclampsia, eclampsia and HELP syndrome are correlated with IUGR. Fetal chromosomal abnormalities also increase the risk of comorbid IUGR.

The two types of intrauterine growth restriction can be distinguished by sonography; they are asymmetric IUGR and symmetric IUGR. Asymmetric IUGR describes an unequal decrease in the size of fetal anatomical structures. In asymmetric IUGR, normal sonographic biparietal diameter measurements may exist, but abdominal circumference measurements may be well below the expected ranges. This is often times due to fetal malnutrition secondary to placental insufficiency. The fetus with asymmetric IUGR will direct its energy to maintaining the heart and brain (thus normal development) at the expensive of the liver and other structures. Symmetrical IUGR is the second type. Symmetrical IUGR reveals proportionate decreased measurements and size in all major fetal structures.

A fetus with asymmetric intrauterine growth restriction is most likely to display signs of compensation secondary to their inadequate nutrition. Fetal compensation occurs in effort to maintain the vital organ of the fetus, the heart and brain. In this case, fetal blood flow and nutrient delivery will be to these organs often times maintaining normal growth and development. However, with all or most of the fetal blood flow and nourishment being directed to the heart and brain, other organs take the loss and lack adequate blood flow, nutrition, and development. Most notable are the liver and kidney. This is often readily apparent on sonography by the middle of the second trimester, which normally sees the most rapid fetal abdominal growth.

Abnormal placentation may be present in a variety of circumstances including placenta previa, placenta abruption, placenta accreta, circumvallate placenta, placental hemangioma, placental infarction, and severe maternal vascular disease. All of these placental abnormalities increase the likelihood of intrauterine growth restriction. Placental malformation leading to intrauterine growth restriction is a direct result of lack of placental oxygenation. Without adequate oxygenation, the placenta cannot provide adequate nutrition to the fetus. This circumstance can be independent of adequate maternal nutrition, especially in the event of placental infarction.

Fetal Macrosomia

Macrosomia is a retrospective diagnosis, meaning it can only be diagnosed upon obtaining the birth weight of a newborn after delivery. Macrosomia refers to a birth weight of greater than 90% expected for gestational age or a birth weight between 8 lb 12 oz and 9 lb 15 oz. Several factors increase the risk for delivering a large-for-age baby including: gestational diabetes, maternal obesity, Hispanic race, excessive maternal weight gain, and male fetus. Cesarean delivery, neonatal and maternal birthing injuries, and neonatal morbidity are common complications associated with fetal macrosomia.

Abnormal Central Nervous System

Agenesis Corpus Callosum

Agenesis of the corpus callosum describes a condition in which the portion of the brain (corpus callosum) that connects the two brain hemispheres is either absent or poorly formed. This condition can be seen independently or with other congenital malformations such as Dandy-Walker and Arnold-Chiari. Sonographic evaluation can identify corpus callosum agenesis between weeks 12 and 18. Associated sonographic changes may include: absent cingulate gyrus, lateral ventricles are further from each other, ventricles appear slightly more vertically positioned when viewing in the coronal plane, and transverse diameter of posterior ventricle is greater than the anterior horn.

Dandy-Walker Malformation

Dandy-Walker malformation is a very rare congenital malformation with variable prognosis. It primarily involves the cerebellum and fourth ventricle of the brain. Dandy-Walker malformation is present when there is an absent or poorly developed cerebellar vermis, cystic fourth ventricle dilation, and posterior fossa enlargement. The diagnosis cannot be made until later in the second trimester. There have been several variants of Dandy-Walker malformation described but all are associated with other fetal defects. Dandy-Walker malformation should be sonographically differentiated from an arachnoid cyst of the posterior fossa. A posterior fossa arachnoid cyst will maintain the presence of the cerebellar vermis and will not be associated with any other fetal malformations.

Schizencephaly, Microcephaly, and Intracranial Calcifications

Schizencephaly is a rare birth defect characterized by slits through the cerebral hemispheres. These abnormal slits can be unilateral or bilateral. Cortical brain matter lines the slits. Microcephaly is a condition in which the fetal head is smaller than expected for gestational age or relative to abdominal circumference and femoral length measurements. Microcephaly is often times associated with other conditions of abnormal brain development. Intracranial calcifications seen in the fetal head with sonography, usually later in pregnancy, may be the result of infection or conditions involving vascular abnormalities/thrombosis.

Hydranencephaly and Porencephaly

Hydranencephaly is a rare condition in which the fetal cerebral hemispheres are completely absent and, in their place, reside cerebrospinal fluid-filled sacs. Sonographic evaluation will reveal an intact falx and meninges. The cerebral cortex is absent or with severe abnormal appearance. If the fetus is delivered, head size, reflexes and general examination may be within normal limits initially. Within the first few weeks of live, changes in muscle tone and development become increasingly apparent. Rarely does an infant born with hydranencephaly survive past the first year of life. Porencephaly is also rare and involves a cystic sac filled with cerebrospinal fluid within the ventricle or subarachnoid space. The sac is lined with white matter. It involves a smaller area than hydranencephaly. Prognosis is dependent on the area of the brain involved and the size of the cyst.

Anencephaly

Anencephaly is a neural tube defect in which the cephalic portion of the neural tube fails to close during development. This stage of closing/development usually happens between the 23rd and 26th days of gestation. The lack of neural tube closure at this stage results in anencephaly, which is marked by an absence of most of the fetal brain, skull, and scalp. The majority of cases of anencephaly are stillborn. Anencephaly is the most common open neural tube defect. If a live birth occurs, survival is not expected much beyond several hours. Although anencephaly develops within the first 4 weeks of gestation, sonographic diagnosis is difficult to make before 10 weeks gestation. Anencephaly is associated with several other fetal anomalies.

Neural Tube Defect

Neural tube defect describes a broad category of developmental birth defects involving the brain and/or spinal cord. Disruption in embryologic closure and formation of the spinal cord and fetal nervous system is responsible for neural tube defects. Neural tube defects are classified according to the type and location of the failed neural tube closure. Neural tube defects develop in the first four gestational weeks, often times before a female is aware of pregnancy. It is thought that at least 400 micrograms of folic acid daily, prior to and during pregnancy can reduce the occurrence of neural tube defects.

Cephaloceles/Encephalocele

When the contents of the cranium protrude through the skull via a defects at a particular region it is termed a cephalocele. Rarely is a cephaloceles an independent fetal defect finding, it is often seen in conjunction with Meckel-Gruber syndrome. Suspect this syndrome in the presence of an occipital cephaloceles, renal dysplasia and in the presence of greater than 5 digits on the hand(s) or foot. When the contents of a cephaloceles include brain tissue, it is termed an encephalocele. Bifid cranium, craniocele, and cranial meningoencephalocele are synonymous with encephalocele. The most common location for an encephalocele is the fronto-orbital and posterior skull region. An encephalocele in the posterior skull is often associated with severe intellectual disability; where as a fronto-orbital encephalocele is less likely to cause intellectual disabilities.

Spina Bifida Occulta and Rachischisis

Spina bifida occulta is the mildest form of spina bifida. It affects up to 10% of the population. It occurs when the neural arch of the vertebra fails to close, but all overlying soft tissue is intact. Therefore, in spina bifida occulta the spinal cord is not exposed or protruding. Obstetrical sonography may not detect spina bifida occulta. X-ray films are usually diagnostic, after delivery. Examination of the newborn may reveal a skin dimple or a tuft of hair growing from the location in the spinal column where the defect exists, usually lumbosacral. Spinal rachischisis is the rarest and most severe form of spina bifida. Spinal rachischisis describes an open spina bifida involving the entire spinal column.

Other Central Nervous System Findings

Dolichocephaly describes a cephalic index of less than 75% and a "long-head" appearance.

Brachycephaly describes a head that appears disproportionately small and has a cephalic index greater than 80%.

Anencephaly is a severe congenital defect in which there is complete absence of the fetal skull, brain, and brainstem.

Holoprosencephaly is a congenital defect in which the forebrain fails to cleave, and a single lobe is present. This is often accompanied by facial defects.

Ventriculomegaly describes a condition in which the fetal lateral brain ventricles are dilated to greater than 10 mm.

Abnormal Intracranial Structures

Cerebral Ventriculomegaly

Mild lateral cerebral ventriculomegaly may also be termed borderline lateral cerebral ventriculomegaly. By definition, this is a slight enlargement of the lateral brain ventricles to an atrial width between 10-15 mm. This condition can be unilateral or bilateral. The cause of this is unknown and its effects range from none to hydrocephalus and other fetal central nervous system defects. If this sonographic finding or diagnosis is present, a thorough search for other fetal defects and associated conditions should be undertaken. Fetal karyotyping should be offered and explained to the mother in this situation.

Ventriculomegaly and Hydrocephaly

Ventriculomegaly is defined as abnormally enlarged lateral ventricles (>15 mm atrial width) in the absence of other central nervous system anomalies on sonography. However, often times other sonographic findings will be associated with ventriculomegaly thus limiting the use of the formal definition. Ventriculomegaly is often seen with hydrocephaly or when the size of the choroid plexus pales next to the size of the ventricle. Hydrocephaly refers to excessive amounts of cerebrospinal fluid often resulting in excess accumulation and dilation of within the ventricles. The presence of hydrocephaly often increases intracranial pressure. However, ventricular enlargement can occur independently of increased intracranial pressure.

Abnormal Face and Neck

Hypotelorism

Hypotelorism is defined as abnormal eye spacing, in which the eyes are abnormally close-set. This condition is usually seen as a result of abnormal or premature fusion of the metopic skull suture. Hypotelorism is seen in conjunction with other brain and facial malformations under the term holoprosencephaly. Hypotelorism can be further divided into subgroups. Cyclopia is its most severe form in which the orbits have fused and there is only a single middle orbit ("cyclops"). Ethmocephaly is a facial formation with abnormally close-set eyes with a proboscis (nose-like protuberance) that starts high above the orbits. Cebocephaly is a form of hypotelorism in which the normally formed and place nasal bridge, but only one nostril is present. The three described forms of hypotelorism are usually associated with fetal mortality.

Cleft Lip and Palate

Cleft lip is a facial abnormality that results when the lateral and median nasal prominences fail to fuse during fetal development. Cleft palate describes a condition in which a fissure develops along the median and anterior palate, also affecting the normal fusion process in fetal development. These terms are often used synonymously, but the conditions can be seen independently or coexist. Cleft palate is further categorized to describe the severity and depth of involvement of the hard palate. The midline cleft may extend to involve the nostrils.

Holoprosencephaly

Holoprosencephaly is a condition in which the fetal brain does not divide normally into two hemispheres. The term also describes a variety of fetal brain and facial defects. There are 4 main types of holoprosencephaly. First is alobar holoprosencephaly describes complete failure of hemispheric division and an absent third ventricle. Second is semilobar holoprosencephaly is partial hemispheric division in the posterior brain with a single ventricular cavity. The third type is lobar holoprosencephaly in which hemispheric division is complete but there is an interhemispheric fissure and some structures may remain fused. The fourth type is the middle interhemispheric variant in which the frontal, posterior and parietal portions of the middle brain are not divided. All forms are usually correlated with a small head and close-set eyes. The prognosis is variable from minimal facial defects and normal intelligence to severe deformity and intellectual disability.

Facial Anomalies

Holoprosencephaly can result in a number of facial defects and anomalies. Close-set eyes (hypotelorism), an abnormally small head (microcephaly), absent incisor teeth, cleft lip and or palate, flat and single nostril (cebocephaly), and multiple nasal deformities are commonly seen in an infant born with holoprosencephaly. Cyclopia (a single midline eye) is another possibility, but this is rare and usually accompanied by the most severe form usually associated with fetal mortality. A dorsal cyst may accompany the diagnosis of holoprosencephaly. This is a space-occupying cyst that often develops in the posterior region, displacing the posterior cerebral hemispheres into the frontal fossa. Holoprosencephaly must be sonographically differentiated from hydranencephaly and hydrocephaly. Both of these conditions maintain a central falx not seen in holoprosencephaly.

Holoprosencephaly, Microphthalmia, and Hypertelorism

Holoprosencephaly is a condition in which the forebrain only develops into a single hemisphere or lobe. This condition is often accompanied with many facial and chromosomal anomalies. In its mildest form, the anterior bony palate does not form causing a cleft palate. This is also known as premaxillary agenesis. The cleft is usually midline on the face and can extend to involve the nostrils. The rest of the face is relatively flat with close-set eyes. Microphthalmia is a condition in which the fetal orbit, and thus the eyes are smaller than normal. Microphthalmia may involve one or both eyes. Hypertelorism is a condition in which the orbits and eyes are further apart than normal. In this condition, the distance between the orbits is greater than the diameter of the orbit itself. In severe cases, the eyes may almost appear on the sides of the face.

Structures Visualized Sonographically in an Abnormal Fetal Neck

The fetal neck is important to evaluate thoroughly during an ultrasound exam to rule out cystic hygromas, goiters, teratomas, hemangiomas, and proximity of the umbilical cord. Diagnosing these anomalies may help improve the mortality rate after birth, and although some have a similar appearance, it is important to try to discern the type. Determining if a mass is cystic, solid, or complex is an advantage of the use of ultrasound during an OB exam. Sonographers should try to determine the size of the mass, where the mass originated from, and if there is an association with other fetal structures. Sometimes even in the presence of abnormalities of the neck, the skull or face may be involved. Color, power, and spectral Doppler are useful to determine the vascularity of these structures.

Cystic Hygroma

A cystic hygroma is created when the lymphatic system cannot effectively drain the lymphatic fluid, causing retention. Cystic hygromas will present as a cyst or multiple cysts on ultrasound. These fluid-filled structures are typically on the posterior or posterolateral portion of the fetal neck, but they can also be found in an anterior location. Often, these cysts contain thick septations that may give the appearance of a mass that is solid. These thick septations can have a similar appearance to a teratoma, but it is important to try to discern between the two. The prognosis for a teratoma can be more promising if they are small. However, a cystic hygroma may give insight to chromosomal malformations that are often present, such as Turner syndrome and trisomies 18 and 21, although these tend to contain more septations and are bigger in Turner syndrome.

Teratoma

Teratomas are masses that are made up of various tissues such as bone, teeth, thyroid tissue, and hair. Because of the multitude of tissues this mass is comprised of, the ultrasound appearance may include solid and cystic components, with many being completely solid. A commonality that may help with a diagnosis of a teratoma is the visualization of calcifications within the mass. Most teratomas are visualized in the lower portion of the spine, but those found in the neck may be located in the thyroid or anterolateral neck regions. The latter may have a similar appearance to a cystic hygroma, but it is important to document the size and origin whenever possible. Color Doppler will often display increased blood flow within the mass. The prognosis in this region, although benign, will often be determined by the patency of the fetal airway.

Goiter

Most fetal thyroid conditions are the result of a maternal thyroid condition, but primary hypothyroidism can occur in a fetus. When mothers have thyroid conditions such as

Hashimoto's thyroiditis or Graves' disease, these antibodies that are produced in the mother can be passed on to the fetus via the placenta. It is important to provide doctors with clinical and diagnostic information about thyroid dysfunction because, if untreated, these conditions may increase neonatal mortality rates. Goiters that are found on OB scans will demonstrate the soft tissues of the neck bulging anteriorly. The thyroid will be enlarged because of the presence of a homogeneous, bilateral mass in the anterior portion of the neck. If these are not a solitary finding, it is typically the result of hyperthyroidism, in which case the fetus may also demonstrate hydrops and a rapid heart rate.

Hemangioma

Hemangiomas, otherwise known as birthmarks, are the most common type of lesion seen in newborns. They are yet another type of tumor that may be visualized during a scan of the fetal head and neck. If a hemangioma can be detected with ultrasound, they typically include bigger vessels that are within the deeper layers of the skin such as the hypodermis and dermis as well as the smaller channels in the epidermis. These will display hypervascularity when color Doppler is used, and they can become quite large. Exophytic hemangiomas may cover the entire neck and face and appear to be a solid mass with an echotexture that resembles the placenta. Follow-up ultrasounds may show an increase in size. Regardless of the type of mass present in the region of the fetal neck, they are important to note because the airway may be compromised at birth.

Micrognathia and Macroglossia

Micrognathia refers to an abnormally small jaw. This is a fetal anomaly often associated with many other fetal syndromes and defects although it can be seen independent of another condition. Micrognathia can correct itself with growth and development. Micrognathia may interfere with normal respiration and feeding early in life and teeth malalignment later on. Macroglossia refers to a condition in which the tongue is larger than normal. Macroglossia is associated with a number of other fetal abnormalities and syndromes. It may be seen on sonography later in gestation. If the fetal tongue repetitively extends beyond the fetal lips on sonographic evaluation, suspect the diagnosis.

Abnormal Fetal Heart

Atrial Ventricular Septal Defects

Septal heart defects are further categorized into atrial or ventricular, thus describing the location in which the defect occurs. Essentially these are a hole in the muscular septal wall that divides the chambers. Ventricular septal defects are difficult to diagnose with routine fetal sonography, especially if the defect is small. Atrial septal defects are also difficult to detect because of the normal fetal blood flow that occurs through the foramen ovale.

Ebstein's Anomaly

Ebstein's anomaly is a congenital heart defect with an abnormal tricuspid valve. This valve is displaced further into the right ventricle. As a result of this displacement, signs of an Ebstein's anomaly may include right ventricular enlargement and pulmonary artery narrowing. It is common for atrial septal defects to coexist with Ebstein's anomaly.

Cardiac Anomalies

The four-chamber view allows for visualization of many structures and since it is usually the easiest and most standardized view to obtain, it allows for detection of a number of anomalies. Among the ventricular anomalies that may be detected with four-chamber viewing are: single ventricle (absence of ventricular septum), atrioventricular canal, poorly developed ventricles, or enlarged ventricles. Four-chamber imaging of the fetal heart may also reveal valvular anomalies such as: absent mitral valve, absent tricuspid valve, and a displaced tricuspid valve (Ebstein's anomaly).

Cardiac Structural Anomalies

Abnormal development or absence of the ventricular septum leads to a rare congenital heart defect of single ventricle. This condition may also be termed univentricular heart. In this condition, the two atria are normal and there may be one or two atrial ventricular valves. Common surgical repair procedures include: Fontan operation, Blalock-Taussig shunting, Glenn shunting, and banding the pulmonary artery. Without surgical intervention, a univentricular heart is not conducive to sustained life. Persistent truncus arteriosus is essentially a large ventricular septal defect often times with a large vessel anomaly in which there is only one ventricular artery. Prenatal diagnosis may be made with sonographic viewing along the long-axis of a large outflow tract and four-chamber view of a ventricular septal defect. These findings would necessitate further evaluation with Doppler studies and fetal echocardiography.

Hypoplastic Left Heart Syndrome

Hypoplastic left heart syndrome is a congenital heart defect in which the entire left side of the heart, including the aorta; aortic valve; left ventricle; and mitral valve are poorly developed. Atrial septal defects and large patent ductus arteriosus are often present with hypoplastic left heart syndrome. Hypoplastic left heart syndrome is responsible for about 8% of all congenital heart defects and is more common in boys. Prenatal diagnosis is more likely with fetal echocardiography.

Coarctation of the Aorta

Coarctation of the aorta is a narrowing of the aorta. It is among the top 3 most common congenital birth defects. It may be an independent finding and condition, but more commonly is seen with other heart defects including: a bicuspid aortic valve, ventricular septal defect, stenosis of the aortic or mitral valve, and patent ductus arteriosus. Routine fetal ultrasound may not detect this condition.

Tetralogy of Fallot

Tetralogy of Fallot is a congenital heart defect comprised of a ventricular septal defect, pulmonary stenosis, an abnormal or overriding aortic valve, and right ventricular hypertrophy. Tetralogy of Fallot is present in up to 6 in 10,000 births. Tetralogy of Fallot may initially be seen as an overriding aorta in the long-axis view on routine fetal heart sonography.

Double-Outlet Right Ventricle

Double-outlet right ventricle is a congenital heart defect in which both the aortic and pulmonic arteries arise from the right ventricle. In the presence of a double-outlet right ventricle is a ventricular septal defect. Short-axis view on routine fetal cardiac sonographic evaluation may best demonstrate this defect initially.

Transposition of Arteries

Transposition of the great arteries is a congenital heart defect in which the aortic artery is connected to the right ventricle (instead of the left ventricle) and the pulmonary artery is connected to the left ventricle (instead of the right ventricle). This transposition compromises the circulation of oxygenated and deoxygenated blood to and from the body.

The "D" in D-transposition refers to dextro-transposition of the great arteries and describes the position of the aortic artery to be anterior and to the right of the pulmonary artery. L-transposition of the great arteries refers to the location of the aortic artery anterior and to the left of the pulmonary artery.

Cardiomyopathy and Atrioventricular Canal Defect

If an enlarged fetal heart is seen on routine fetal sonography, further detail and measurements should be obtained, as this is a sign of fetal cardiomyopathy. The heart chambers themselves may be larger or the muscular septum and heart walls may be thickened causing the enlargement. Note must be made if this is diffuse thickening and enlargement or localized to a single heart chamber. Atrioventricular canal defect is a condition in which the mitral and tricuspid valves do not form normally and individually and a single defect/hole/valve forms that communicates between the atrium and ventricles. This is usually readily seen in routine fetal heart sonography. Sonographically, AVC is seen as a gooseneck deformity with left ventricular outflow narrowing. Doppler studies are then needed to estimate the degree of defect.

Echocardiography and Cardiac Abnormalities

Congenital heart defects are present in up to 1 in every 100 births, thus necessitating advanced imaging techniques. Fetal echocardiography allows for a detailed assessment of the fetal heart structure and function. The use and application of fetal echocardiography is well documented. Fetal echocardiograms are a relatively non-invasive and low- to no-risk procedure; even so, they are not currently recommended for routine screening. Fetal echocardiography allows for early diagnosis of a wide variety of congenital heart defects; furthermore, early detection of defects allows for management plans in utero or during and after delivery.

Since fetal echocardiography is not currently a standard screening procedure, guidelines have been established for those that should undergo it. Certainly, if there is a family history of congenital heart disease the fetal heart should be evaluated with echocardiography. Maternal conditions such as type I diabetes, early drug or chemical exposure (some seizure medications and illegal drugs), and infections should warrant a fetal echocardiogram. An abnormal amniocentesis, fetal arrhythmia, or abnormal fetal heart structure are indications for fetal echocardiography. If routine obstetrical sonography detects abnormal amniotic fluid amounts, fetal situs inversus, decreased fetal size, 2-vessel umbilical cord, or the absence of a fetal spleen echocardiography should be considered.

Pentalogy of Cantrell

As its name suggests, the pentalogy of Cantrell is a rare disorder characterized by five fetal defects. The five defects are: abdominal wall defect, lower sternum defect, diaphragmatic hernia, pericardium defect, and intracardiac defects. This pentad of defects develops around the 6th – 7th gestational week, with abnormal abdominal mesoderm folding. In half of the cases, an atrial septal defect will be present. A number of noncardiac fetal defects are also associated with this condition. Sonographically, the heart will appear exposed or outside of the thorax and omphalocele will be present.

Abnormal Thorax

Pulmonary Hypoplasia and Pleural Effusions

Pulmonary hypoplasia may develop if optimal fetal lung development conditions are not present. Among the conditions that might impair the normal development are: inadequate thoracic space secondary to mass or effusion, abnormal fetal breathing, abnormal amniotic fluid volume, and deficient fetal production of lung fluid and surfactant. An insufficient thoracic space may be diagnosed if it is significantly smaller than the fetal abdominal circumference. Fetal pleural effusion can be a primary or secondary condition occurring in one or both fetal lungs. The prevalence of fetal pleural effusion is approximated at 1 in every 15,000 pregnancies.

Pulmonary Sequestration

Pulmonary sequestration is further termed extralobar sequestration to describe a condition that develops in the fetus or neonate. Extralobar pulmonary sequestration is marked by the development of abnormal cystic lung tissue that does not have any connection to the tracheobronchial tree. Furthermore, this anomalous area receives its blood supply from the abdominal aorta rather than the pulmonary artery. Extralobar pulmonary sequestration can be seen in as many as 6% of all congenital thoracic anomalies. Prognosis is good in most cases. Diagnosis may be prenatal with Doppler studies or more often postnatal with a variety of work-ups leading to the diagnosis and extent.

Cystic Adenomatoid Malformations

Cystic adenomatoid malformations (CAM) in the fetal lung are unilateral and broken into three subtypes: cystic, cystic and solid, and solid. CAM develops when an abnormal cystic tissue of the lung develops and occupies a large portion of where the normal lung should be. It can occur in either lung equally and over all prevalence is unclear but estimated at 1 in every 30,000 pregnancies with a slight male over female predominance. CAM is responsible for about 25% of all congenital pulmonary lesions. Sonographically, CAM may be diagnosed by a highly echogenic mass in the fetal thorax with cardiac displacement and a flat or everted diaphragm.

Tracheal Atresia and Bronchogenic Cysts

Fetal tracheal atresia is the absence of a normal or patent tracheal opening and is a very rare finding. Sonographically, the fetal lungs appear enlarged and hyperechogenic as a result of dilated alveoli. The heart will appear relatively small in the midline. Tracheal atresia is most common at the level of the larynx and is often associated with other fetal anomalies. Bronchogenic cysts are a rare condition that may result during fetal bronchi development later in pregnancy. The diagnosis is not usually made prenatally. The location rather than the size of the bronchogenic cysts determine outcome, with bronchogenic cysts at the carina being the most severe and life threatening.

Situs Abnormalities, Cardiac Tumors and Rhythm Abnormalities

Situs inversus, also called situs transverses, is a condition in which the abdominal and/or thoracic contents are reversed. If only the heart is involved (located on the right side) it is termed dextrocardia. Care must be taken in imaging these individuals, with special attention to landmarks, positioning, and labeling "left" and "right". Fetal cardiac tumors are an extremely rare finding. When they are present, about 90% of them are benign. The most common benign cardiac tumor is a rhabdomyoma. Fetal sonography may detect the mass, but cannot differentiate tumor-type. Evaluation of fetal heart rate is important, as up to 2% of all fetuses have an arrhythmia. Many of these resolve spontaneously. Normal fetal heart rates range from 120 – 180 beats per minute. If irregularities are sonographically detected, the duration, frequency and type of irregularity should be documented and followed.

Congenital Diaphragmatic Hernia

Congenital diaphragmatic hernia (CDH) occurs as frequently as 1 in every 2,500 live births. Diaphragmatic herniation occurs from failure of diaphragmatic structures to fuse normally be the 10th gestational week. CDH more frequently involves the left diaphragm. The prognosis is based on the area of herniation and the abdominal contents that have herniated. Sonographic evaluation of a diaphragmatic hernia will likely reveal fetal heart displacement to the right side of the thorax. Abdominal contents such as the bowel, stomach, and even the liver, may be seen in the thoracic cavity. The presence of a congenital diaphragmatic hernia is highly correlated with trisomy 18 and its associated anomalies.

Abnormal Abdomen

Omphalocele

An omphalocele is the herniation of fetal abdominal contents (usually intestine) through the umbilical cord opening, with the development of these contents outside of the fetal abdominal cavity. A thin membrane covers the ruptured abdominal contents. The incidence of omphalocele is similar to that of gastroschisis. Omphalocele has a high percentage of associated fetal and chromosomal anomalies. Common chromosomal anomalies associated with omphalocele are trisomy 18, 13, and 21. Common fetal anomalies associated with omphalocele are a number of cardiac defects. Diagnosis is with AFP testing and ultrasound findings. Prognosis for omphalocele is dependent of the extent of the secondary anomalies.

Gastroschisis

Gastroschisis is a condition in which fetal abdominal contents herniate through an opening in the abdominal wall, usually to the right of the fetal umbilical cord. Gastroschisis occurs in up to 2.5 per 1000 births and in slightly more males than females. In most cases of gastroschisis, the nonrotated small intestine is the only structure that herniates through the abdominal wall. Rarely will the liver, stomach or colon protrude through the opening. The exact mechanisms and risks for development of gastroschisis are unknown, but many theories involve obstruction of the omphalomesenteric vessels. Prenatal diagnosis with sonography and AFP testing is common. Associated fetal anomalies are rare, and usually are related to the defect itself. With increased technology and surgical repair methods, survival is up to 90%.

Limb-Body Wall Complex

Limb-body wall complex (LBWC), also known as body stalk anomaly, is a rare birth defect occurring approximately once for every 10,000 pregnancies. Limb-body wall complex is primarily characterized by a severe abdominal wall defect, prominent kyphoscoliosis, and a poorly developed umbilical cord. A number of other defects may be present including, but not limited to, cranial and facial defects and limb anomalies. Forty percent of body stalk anomalies also have the presence of amniotic bands. The exact etiology of limb-body wall complex is unknown. Sonographically, the liver may appear attached to the placenta. Sonographic imaging of the umbilical cord may reveal its absence or a poorly developed and abnormally short umbilical cord. Significant spinal distortion will be present and, if identified, the limbs will be grossly abnormal. Body stalk anomalies are always fatal.

Evaluating Abdominal Wall Defects

In obstetrical sonography, evaluation of fetal abdominal wall defects is important to identify independent anomalies as well as defects that are correlated with additional fetal anomalous conditions. The first sonographic protocol is to establish abdominal landmarks, specifically in relation to the umbilical cord. Second, sonography needs to establish if a membranous material covers the defect, and this needs to be thoroughly described. Third, identify the fetal organ structures that are involved in the defect and to what extent. Fourth, if the abdominal defect involves fetal bowel, sonographic differentiation of stricture or dilation needs to be noted. Finally, with the presence of any sonographic fetal abdominal wall defect, thorough investigation, imaging, and description of all other areas of fetal, uterine and placenta anatomy need to be noted.

Cloacal Exstrophy

Cloacal exstrophy is a rare set of birth anomalies occurring about once in every 250,000 live births. It is also known as OEIS complex, which better describes the set of anomalies that are present: Omphalocele, Exstrophy of the cloaca (open bladder with rectal communication), Imperforate anus, and Spinal defects (especially spina bifida). Diagnosis of cloacal exstrophy is with elevated AFP tests and sonograph. Sonographically, the OEIS complex will reveal a tissue mass inferior to the fetal umbilicus attachment site, a fluid-filled mass in the pelvis (cloaca), and often times the absence of the anterior pelvic bones. Due to prenatal diagnostic techniques, survival rate is improved but will likely result in a number of postnatal surgical procedures. Probable postnatal surgeries include: repair of omphalocele; repair of bladder and rectum/anus (creating bowel and bladder elimination routes), and often times surgical sexual determination and repair (males will be surgically made female, and females will have surgical vagina created).

Beckwith-Wiedemann Syndrome

Beckwith-Wiedemann syndrome is a congenital disorder marked by larger-than-expected body and organ size. Often omphalocele and asymmetric fetal limbs are characteristic of Beckwith-Wiedemann syndrome. Up to 80% of cases involve a defect on chromosome number 11. The diagnosis of Beckwith-Wiedemann syndrome is usually made in infancy by a number of findings including: hypoglycemia, enlarged fontanelle, x-ray of long bones, abdominal CT scan, and testing for defects on chromosome 11. The prognosis for Beckwith-Wiedemann syndrome is variable. Individuals with this disorder are at increased risk for tumor development. If the survive infancy, prognosis is improved.

Abnormal Gastrointestinal System

Esophageal Atresia

Esophageal atresia is a congenital disorder in which the esophagus does not develop normally. There are several types of esophageal atresia, but two common conditions are: the failure of the upper esophagus to connect to its inferior portion and thus the stomach, and a fistula that develops between the esophagus and trachea. It is difficult to detect this directly with prenatal sonography, but in the presence of increased amniotic fluid and other congenital anomalies (cardiac, renal, limb, vertebral, and anal), esophageal atresia should be highly suspected. Prognosis is based on early detection and the extent of other anomalies.

Colon Atresia

Colon atresia accounts for up to 10% of intestinal bowel atresias. Most colon atresias are secondary to vascular or nerve injury to the affected colonic portion. Colon atresia is not associated with increased amniotic fluid findings and may first be suspected or diagnosed in the third trimester when the colonic diameter exceeds 18 mm. The most common colon atresia is anorectal atresia, which is associated with cardiac, kidney, limb, vertebral, and upper GI tract anomalies. Colon atresia often coexists with a more proximal small bowel atresia. If not diagnosed before birth, the first signs of colonic atresia will be the absence of infant bowel movements, abdominal distention and vomiting.

Duodenal Atresia

Duodenal atresia refers to a condition in which the duodenum is closed and does not allow for passage of stomach contents into the small intestines. The incidence of duodenal atresia is 1 in 10,000 births. Rarely is duodenal atresia an independent finding. Thirty percent are also associated with Down syndrome. Sonographically, duodenal atresia may be suspected and diagnosed with increased amniotic fluid and swollen stomach and proximal duodenum (double bubble sign), often seen after 24 gestational weeks. With early diagnosis and surgical repair, prognosis is good. Undetected and untreated duodenal atresia is fatal.

Echogenic Small Bowel

Echogenic small bowel, if present, is usually seen in the second trimester ultrasound. Sonographically, the bowel is hyperechogenic and brighter than the nearest fetal bone. Echogenic small bowel may be seen after amniocentesis if the fetus swallows bloody amniotic fluid. The presence of echogenic small bowel raises the possibility of a fetus with cystic fibrosis, as this finding is present in up to 80% of these fetuses. Echogenic small bowel is also highly correlated with several chromosomal anomalies. Echogenic small bowel may be the result of any number of congenital infections. There is increased likelihood of late pregnancy fetal demise in the presence of hyperechoic small bowel.

Meconium Ileus and Peritonitis

Meconium ileus is a condition in which the ileus portion of the small intestine fills with meconium causing an obstruction and/or dilation of the ileum at this point. With this finding, the colon will be smaller than expected for gestational age or may not be visualized at all. The presence of meconium ileus is highly correlated with cystic fibrosis. Meconium peritonitis is the result of perforated intestine/colon in utero. The intestinal contents (bowel and meconium) then leak into the abdominal/peritoneal cavity. Sonographic appearance of meconium peritonitis reveals hyperechogenic areas and punctate and linear calcifications throughout the fetal abdomen.

Abnormal Genitourinary System

Fetal Bladder Outlet Obstruction

Fetal bladder obstruction can be detected as early as 12 weeks gestation by ultrasound. Sonographic and diagnostic findings include insufficient amniotic fluid, hydronephrosis, echogenic kidneys, pelvic diameter greater than 4mm, and an enlarged fetal urinary bladder. the most common cause of lower urinary tract obstruction in a fetus is the presence of posterior urethral valves. This is seen in as many as 1 in 5000 male fetuses, with a mortality rate as high as 63%. With these occurrence and mortality rates, the search for definitive treatments and urinary bladder decompression methods has been sought. Several in utero procedures have been attempted, usually during the second trimester and usually and involve some sort of catheter placement or various shunting methods. Many fetal bladder decompression techniques have been limited by device dislodgement, short functional life, and obstruction.

Hydronephrosis

Hydronephrosis refers to enlargement of the fetal kidney secondary to urine back up from an outlet anomaly. This condition may be unilateral or bilateral. Sonographically, a dilated ureter may be seen in addition to the swollen kidney. Sonographically, the fetal kidney and bladder can be seen as early as 15 weeks gestation. By about 18 weeks, the renal sinus can be seen as a central echo. If the anterior to posterior kidney measurement of the renal pelvis is greater than 8 mm by the 20th gestational week or 10 mm after 20 weeks gestation, the diagnosis of hydronephrosis can be made. Hydronephrosis is the most common fetal anomaly detected, and account for about half of all genitourinary anomalies. Rarely is hydronephrosis and independent diagnosis, rather a symptom of another disorder. Prognosis is dependent upon pregnancy stage, unilateral or bilateral kidney involvement, and degree of kidney swelling/ureter dilation.

Urethral Obstruction and Prune Belly Syndrome

Urethral obstruction appears sonographically as an enlarged renal pelvis, a dilated and/or twisted ureter, and a thickened bladder wall. In the male fetus, the most likely site of ureter obstruction is in the posterior urethral valves. In the female fetus, urethral obstruction is usually secondary to a cloacal anomaly. In cases of complete and severe urethral obstruction, the renal tissue will develop abnormally giving the kidneys a cystic or echogenic appearance. Prune belly syndrome, also known as Eagle-Barrett syndrome is a rare set of birth defects seen in the male fetus. Prune belly syndrome is characterized by absence of abdominal wall musculature, hydronephrosis, hydroureters, enlarged urinary bladder and undescended testes.

Ureteropelvic Junction Obstruction, Ureterovesical Junction Obstruction, and Pyelectasis

Ureteropelvic junction obstruction (UPJ) is a condition in which there is a blockage at the junction of the renal pelvis and the ureter. This obstruction is manifest by kidney enlargement. It is more common in the male fetus. Ureterovesical junction obstruction (UVJ) or reflux may be seen with sonography of the fetal kidney when both the renal pelvis and the ureter are enlarged. Sonography is unable to differentiate obstruction versus reflux at this site. This finding is more common in the female fetus. Pyelectasis refers to the mildest form of hydronephrosis or enlarged renal pelvis of the kidney. Pyelectasis is seen as an independent finding in about 1% of chromosomal anomalies and in 2% of normal fetuses. Pyelectasis is found in up to 25% of fetuses with trisomy 21.

Renal Cystic Disease

Renal cystic diseases, also known as Potter's syndromes, are classified into four disease types using six criteria. The renal cystic disease type classification uses the Roman numeral system and labels the four types as: Potter's Type I, Potter's Type II, and etc. However, it is the first criteria of nomenclature type that probably best describes each of the four renal cystic disease classifications. The second and third classification criteria are based on location and sonographic appearance. The fourth criterion evaluates the volume of amniotic fluid associated with each type of renal cystic disease. The fifth classification criterion is based on outcome or prognosis. And finally, the sixth classification criterion labels the risk of a fetus having renal cystic disease in future pregnancies.

Potter's Type I

Potter's Type I, better described as autosomal recessive polycystic kidney disease (ARPKD), is a rare and often fatal form of renal cystic disease. ARPKD usually involves both fetal kidneys and there is usually an insufficient amount of amniotic fluid during pregnancy. Sonographically, the kidneys will be enlarged with multiple cysts. Centrally, the kidney is echogenic with hypoechoic borders. If a hypoechoic halo of cortical tissue borders the kidney, this finding is diagnostic. Often biliary duplication cysts and liver defects are associated with Potter's Type I kidney disease. Close sonographic evaluation of the entire fetal development is necessary, as several other conditions may have similar kidney findings, especially Meckel-Gruber syndrome and trisomy 13.

Potter's Type II

Multicystic dysplastic kidney disease (Potter's Type II) is a condition in which the kidney(s) contain multiple cysts, may be of varying size, and echogenic. Both kidneys can be involved, but unilateral involvement is more common, bilateral involvement carries a poor prognosis. Sonographic diagnosis may be difficult until the second trimester. In Potter's Type II kidney disease, the cysts do not communicate like they would in hydronephrosis. Multicystic dysplastic kidney disease is thought to arise from an early obstruction. Males are more likely to develop unilateral Potter's Type II, females are more likely to develop bilateral multicystic dysplastic kidney.

Potter's Type III and IV

Autosomal dominant polycystic kidney disease (Potter's Type III) is primarily an adult-onset disorder that usually affects both kidneys. In the rare cases that it would be seen on fetal ultrasound, multiple cysts formation will be noted in the kidneys as well as other organ structures such as the liver, pancreas and spleen. Potter's Type IV or obstructive renal dysplasia classification system is largely dependent on the underlying cause of the obstruction. In many cases it is secondary to obstruction at the ureteropelvic junction and posterior urethral valves. Sonographically, cysts will be apparent but the renal pyramid(s) will not be visualized.

Unilateral Renal Agenesis and Renal Ectopia

Unilateral renal agenesis is a condition in which the fetus only develops one functional kidney. This condition is compatible with life. Sonographically, a normal appearing fetal kidney will be present as well as a normal urinary bladder and adequate amniotic fluid. In the space of the absent kidney will be the elongated and flattened adrenal gland. Renal ectopia describes a condition in which one or both kidneys are positioned outside of the normal renal fossa. The kidney(s) may be positioned anywhere from the chest to the pelvis and are often malrotated. Occurrence is 1 in 1,000 births but only 1 of every 10 of them is diagnosed, usually as an incidental finding. If discovered, evaluate for other congenital abnormalities.

Bilateral Renal Agenesis

Bilateral renal agenesis is a genetic disorder in which the fetal kidneys fail to develop. This occurs in up to 1 in every 4000 births. In the absence of fetal kidneys, there is most definitely oligohydramnios. With insufficient amniotic cushioning, several other defects follow: limb contractures, flattening nose, low-set ears, bell-shaped thorax, and even sirenomelia. Further sonographic evaluation will reveal an elongated, flattened, and echogenic adrenal gland in the absence of no pelvic kidney or urinary bladder. Bilateral renal agenesis is always fatal ultimately secondary to hypoplastic formation of the pulmonary system.

Meckel-Gruber Syndrome

Meckel-Gruber syndrome is always a fatal condition primarily due to its severe polycystic kidney disease and malformation. In addition to the dysplastic kidney, an encephalocele may develop, and liver and lung malformations are great enough that they cannot support life. Polydactyly, facial, and genital defects may be noted secondarily. Insufficient amniotic fluid will always be present with Meckel-Gruber syndrome. Meckel-Gruber syndrome is rare and does not have a male or female predominance. It is genetic and both parents must have contributed their recessive gene of with the defect for the fetus to develop Meckel-Gruber syndrome.

Neuroblastoma and Congenital Mesoblastic Nephroma

A neuroblastoma is a malignant tumor of embryonic nerve cells. A neuroblastoma can occur anywhere but about 30% of them are associated with the adrenal gland. Prenatal diagnosis may be difficult, but may appear sonographically as a mass invading the fetal kidney. Congenital mesoblastic nephroma is usually diagnosed postnatally as an abdominal or renal mass finding. It is the most common renal tumor of infancy, with greater than 60% being diagnosed in the first 3 months of life and 90% diagnosed by 1 year of age. They generally do not metastasize but can become large enough to invade surrounding tissue and compromise other organ functions. Removal is curative.

Hydrocele, Cryptorchidism, and Hydrometrocolpos

A hydrocele refers to a collection of serous fluid within the scrotum, surrounding the testes. In the developing fetus it may be a sign of a developmental anomaly or in a worst-case scenario one developing fetal hydrops. Hydroceles are correlated with increase inguinal herniation. Cryptorchidism is the failure of one or both testes to descend from the pelvis/abdomen after 30 weeks gestation. This is commonly termed undescended testes. This may be an independent finding or associated with other anomalies. Hydrometrocolpos is a condition found in females in which excessive mucous secretions collect in the genitourinary tract, especially the uterus and vagina. Hydrometrocolpos and imperforate hymen are often used interchangeably.

Fetal Genital Malformations

Fetal genital malformation possibilities are numerous. They may be secondary to a chromosomal disorder or originate from improper embryonic development, closure and fusion. Defective genital formation affects both male and female fetuses and can result in ambiguous male/female. Adrenal hyperplasia can also result in fetal genital malformation. Many genital defects occur between the 12th and 16th gestational weeks, as this is the normal time in which differentiation occurs. Examples of male genital malformations are: penile agenesis and duplication, penile torsion, microphallus, scrotal agenesis, and penoscrotal transposition. Examples of female genital defects are: ectopic labium, labial adhesions, clitoral duplication, clitoral hypertrophy, and interlabial masses.

Abnormal Skeletal System

Short-Limb Skeletal Dysplasia

Short-limb skeletal dysplasia, also known as dwarfism, refers to a group of disorders in which the fetus develops a disproportionate short skeletal stature and limbs. There are several sub-groups of skeletal dysplasia, many dependent on when in the gestational age that the skeletal development becomes abnormal. A short stature is generally defined as any height measurements that are greater than 3 standard deviations below those expected for age. The true incidence of skeletal dysplasia is difficult to determine because many diagnoses are made well into childhood, but incidence is estimated at 1 in every 4000 births. If marked sonographic evidence of skeletal dysplasia occurs before the 20th gestational week, the prognosis is poor and the fatality rate is high.

If short-limb skeletal dysplasia is suspected in the fetus, thorough sonographic examination, description and measurements in a number of areas are needed. When measuring the extremities and long bones (including hands and feet), it is important to differentiate whether shortening occurs in the proximal segment (rhizomelic), middle segment (mesomelic), distal segment (acromelic), middle and distal segments (acromesomelic), or all three segments (micromelia). This helps identify the type of short-limb dysplasia. Fetal skull measurement, shape, flexibility, density, and ossification need to be noted. Sonographic detail of the fetal skeletal thorax should be obtained including notes on circumference at various levels and symmetry. The fetal spine imaging should include detail on the ossification of the vertebrae. Finally, note any facial anomalies that may be present to help with the diagnosis of the type and extent of skeletal dysplasia present.

Thanatophoric Dwarfism

Thanatophoric dwarfism is the most common lethal skeletal dysplasia. The prevalence is estimated at 1 in every 25,000 live births. Classic sonographic characteristics of thanatophoric dwarfism are marked micromelia in all limbs, megacephaly, and reduced thorax circumference but with a normal length. Thanatophoric dwarfism is further broken down into two types with many overlapping features; however, probably the most obvious differentiator is in type I the skull normally shaped and in type II the skull is a cloverleaf shape. Sonographic diagnosis is usually made in the late second or third trimester. Other sonographic possibilities (type undifferentiated) are: curved “telephone receiver” long bones, especially the femur; extremely short and straight proximal long bones; short ribs; protuberant abdomen; polyhydramnios; flat nasal bridge; proptotic eyes; hydrocephalus; and an average term length of < 40 cm. The presence of polydactyly suggests another type of skeletal dysplasia and is never seen in thanatophoric dwarfism.

Camptomelic Dysplasia, Osteogenesis Imperfecta, and Metatropic Dysplasia

Camptomelic dysplasia is a rare congenital disorder secondary to a mutated gene on chromosome 17. Sonographically, camptomelic dysplasia is marked by severe bilateral bowing of the long bones especially those of the femur and tibia. The curvature and angulation is so great that it may be mistaken for a fracture. Those with camptomelic dysplasia often have clubfeet and prominent occiput and there is a moderate association with ambiguous genitalia. Osteogenesis imperfecta is a set of disorders in which the collagen is either deficient in quantity, quality or both. In its mildest form, osteogenesis imperfecta is conducive to survival. It may also be known as brittle bone syndrome. Mild forms of osteogenesis imperfecta may not be identifiable in utero. Metatropic dysplasia is extremely rare, but can be diagnosed prenatally via characteristic ultrasound findings. Characteristic findings of this short-limbed dysplastic disorder are dumbbell-shaped long bones and a coccygeal appendage or tail.

Osteogenesis Imperfecta Type II

Osteogenesis imperfecta type II is the most severe form of the said class of skeletal dysplasia. Osteogenesis imperfecta type II is caused be a gene mutation that affects collagen formation. Sonographically, this disorder is characterized by crumpled, fragmented, and/or fractured skeletal bones in utero. The fetal thorax is narrow and small, thus affecting lung development. Extremities appear short and bowed. Skull bones are thin, soft, and flexible. Osteogenesis imperfecta type II is not compatible with life, and those with this disorder are either stillborn or succumb shortly after birth from respiratory failure.

Achondrogenesis

Achondrogenesis is a rare skeletal dysplasia that is almost always fatal. The overall incidence is estimated at 1 in 40,000. Achondrogenesis is broken down into type I and type II, with type I being more severe and least compatible with life. Polyhydramnios, breech presentation and hydrops may be present with achondrogenesis. Sonographic characteristics of type I include: extreme micromelia, appendages are "flipper-like", short neck, short and barrel-shaped thorax, protuberant abdomen, cardiac defects, and an average birth weight of 1200 g. Type I is associated with multiple craniofacial anomalies including: microcephaly, soft skull, flat nasal bridge with horizontal groove, small nose with anteverted nostrils, sloping forehead, and overall convexity of facial plane. Type II sonographic findings include many of the same craniofacial, neck, and abdominal findings. Micromelia is present, but to a lesser degree in type II. Birth weight is slightly greater at 2100 g and the thorax is bell-shaped in type II achondrogenesis.

Heterozygous Achondroplasia

Heterozygous achondroplasia is a skeletal condition in which cartilaginous development of the long bones was disrupted. It is an autosomal dominant trait that is not fatal. However, up to 90% of cases are sporadic, which suggests the possibility of a mutation cause of transmission. It is characterized by rhizomelic shortened limbs and a normal thorax. Frontal bossing, trident hands, thoracolumbar kyphosis, and midfacial hypoplasia are common findings and characteristics of heterozygous achondroplasia. Prenatal, sonographic diagnosis is difficult and rare unless one of the parents has achondroplasia.

Polydactyly Syndrome and Hypophosphatasia

Short-rib polydactyly syndrome is a rare and always fatal skeletal dysplasia. Diagnosis is usually made prenatally by the presence of key sonographic features. Key sonographic findings in short-rib polydactyly syndrome include: macrocephaly, poorly-formed and low-set ears, cleft palate and lip, atrophied or bifid tongue, severely reduced and bell-shaped thorax, thick umbilical cord (>3.5 cm), micromelia, and polydactyly usually in the toes. Lethal hypophosphatasia is a rare, inherited metabolic skeletal dysplasia with estimated occurrence at 1 in 100,000. Sonographic features may include: micromelia with metaphyses cupping, significant variability and alternating of bone ossification, short and fragmented ribs, and butterfly-shaped vertebral bodies.

Radial Ray, Clubfoot, and Focal Femoral Hypoplasia

A radial ray anomaly refers to one in which there is a congenital absence of the radius and thumb. This congenital anomaly may be an independent finding or associated with a number of other conditions. A radial ray anomaly may be bilateral or unilateral. In the absence of the radius and thumb, the four fingers project perpendicular to the ulna. Clubfoot is a relatively common (up to 7 in 1000 births) anomaly found independently or in association with other disorders. Clubfoot is an anomaly in which the foot/feet are plantarflexed, adducted and inverted. Focal femoral hypoplasia refers to a usually independent birth anomaly of unilateral or bilateral femoral shortening. This is more common in females and correlated with maternal diabetes.

Spina Bifida Operta

Open spina bifida refers to a defect caused by a failure of the fetal vertebrae to fuse and create a protective column for the spinal cord. Instead, the spinal cord is left exposed and sometimes can protrude. In spina bifida operta, the skin in this area does not come together either, and often the only barrier for the spinal cord to the environment is a thin meningeal membrane. This defect occurs within the first 5 gestational weeks. However, sonography may not detect spina bifida operta until later in pregnancy. Open spina bifida usually occurs in the lumbosacral region.

OTHER SONOGRAPHIC FINDINGS OF THE FETAL SKELETON

Hypertrophic cardiomyopathy describes a condition in which the muscle of the left heart ventricle is thickened, particularly the septal wall. This condition is seen in many congenital defects and is thought to be responsible for sudden cardiac death in athletes.

Hyperplasia describes the presence of increased cellular number in any organ or tissue.

Hyperemesis gravidarum describes severe vomiting or 'morning sickness' of pregnancy.

Hypertelorism describes an abnormally increased distance between two anatomical structures.

Supine hypotensive syndrome describes a condition seen in the third trimester, in which the gravid uterus presses on the inferior vena cava. This may result in decreased venous return in the mother, and fetal hypoxia.

Asynclitism is used to describe any condition in which there is an absence of parallelism or symmetry of anatomical structures.

Anasarca is used to describe any anatomical area of connective tissue that becomes infiltrated with edematous fluid.

Ascites describes a collection of serous fluid localized within the peritoneal region.

Sirenomelia describes a congenital defect in which the legs are fused together, usually with the feet remaining unfused. Also known as "mermaid legs or deformity".

Hygroma is used to describe any increase or swelling in cystic collection of serous fluid.

Polydactyly describes a congenital defect in which there are greater than five digits on a hand(s) or foot (feet). The extra digit(s) usually are comprised of soft tissue only, but may contain bone.

Talipes is used to define any number of congenital anomalies involving the ankle/foot region. One of the more common uses of this term is talipes equinovarus, which is the medical term for 'clubfoot'.

Clinodactyly describes radial or ulnar deviation of the finger digits. This is a congenital anomaly.

Hypospadias is a male congenital defect in which the urethral opening is located more proximal and ventral on the penis, then its normal position.

Macrosomia, also known as 'big baby syndrome', describes a fetus that is large for gestational age (>90th percentile).

Placental and Umbilical Abnormalities

Placental Grading

Placental grading is all but an obsolete practice in modern medicine. Its remaining and rare usage is in describing the appearance of a Grade III or mature placenta too early in pregnancy. This may signal fetal abnormalities. Initially, placental grading was formulated to determine lung maturity of the fetus based on sonographic appearance of the placenta. Increased technology and testing parameters have determined that fetal lung maturity and placental appearance do not correlate well. Grades are given 0 through III. Grade 0 represents a uniform placenta with a smooth chorionic plate. Each successive grade describes increasing echogenic calcifications, densities and cysts.

Placenta Previa

Placenta previa is a condition in which the placenta is abnormally located in relation to the cervical os. Complete placenta previa is defined as a complete coverage of the cervical os by the placenta. Partial placenta previa is described when the border of the placenta covers only a portion of the cervical os. Marginal placenta previa is diagnosed if the placental margin is directly adjacent to the cervical os, but not covering the os. A low-lying placenta previa is described if any portion of the placenta is located near, but not directly adjacent to, the cervical os.

Implications of Placenta Previa, Occurrence Rates, and Causes

The dangers of placenta previa lie in the fact that the placenta is blocking the baby's exit during delivery. As the cervical os dilates and the cervix thins, during labor, the vessels of the placenta may stretch and tear. This causes life-threatening blood loss for both the mother and baby. Reported incidence with which placenta previa occurs varies greatly, from approximately one in every 200 pregnancies to one in every 500 pregnancies. Exact causes of developing placenta previa are unknown, but several risk factors exist. Multiparous women, multiple pregnancy, adhesions, smoking, maternal age greater than 35 years, drug use, and placenta previa in previous pregnancy increase the risk of placenta previa.

Vaginal bleeding is the main sign of placenta previa. This can occur as spotting in the first or second trimester and as profuse and sudden bleeding in the third trimester. Once bleeding is present, cramping may develop but is rare. Blood loss is usually maternal in origin, so signs of fetal distress are usually not apparent initially, but it is important to watch for signs of maternal shock with large amounts of blood loss. Diagnosis of placenta previa is via ultrasound. Ultrasound allows for a precise description of the placental location, especially its relative location to the cervical os. The diagnosis should not be made before 20 weeks of gestation because of normal placental migration and localization. If placenta previa is suspected, digital pelvic exam should be avoided.

Placental Abruption

Placental abruption is the premature separation of the placenta from the uterine wall. This deprives the fetus of nutrients and oxygen and can cause maternal bleeding. The condition can be partial or complete and may be life-threatening to mother and baby. Signs and symptoms are similar to that of placenta previa but usually with greater pain and cramping symptoms. Ultrasound has little value in the diagnosis of placental abruption, and is primarily used to exclude placenta previa. Diagnosis is primarily clinical and with fetal monitoring. Hypertension is the most common cause of abruptio placentae.

Placental Infarction

It is unusual to identify a placental infarction with ultrasound because they are often isoechoic to the placenta, and this can create difficulty in identifying them sonographically. Typically, most placental infarctions involve a minuscule portion of the placenta (less than 5%) and they do not affect the pregnancy. However, if a third or more of the placenta is affected, there is an increased chance of pregnancy complications including premature labor, intrauterine growth restriction, or possibly fetal demise. Placental infarctions are not generally visualized during a sonogram except when a hemorrhage is present, which tends to display a hypoechoic region surrounded by a hyperechoic rim. It has been determined that most infarctions are due to thrombosis of an artery connecting the placenta to the uterus, but some cases are due to hypertension and a pregnancy that has extended beyond the expected due date.

Benefit of Superb Microvascular Imaging If Infarction Is Suspected

Superb microvascular imaging (SMI) is a new ultrasound technology that can detect blood flow that is moving at an extremely slow rate, which includes blood flow within tiny vessels. Often, these small vessels cannot be detected by conventional color or power Doppler imaging. SMI shows promise during OB exams in which a placental infarction is suspected. An infarction cannot typically be visualized sonographically because it appears isoechoic to the surrounding tissue of the placenta (unless it has a hemorrhagic component that appears hypoechoic). SMI is effective at detecting lower velocities because it removes the artifacts created by tissue motion. In a normal placenta, SMI can accurately portray the vessels that branch out to the peripheral villous components in the maternal surface. In cases of placental infarction, this demonstration of branching vessels cannot be visualized with SMI. SMI is also helpful because operators can increase the frame rate to help compensate for a fetus that is moving.

Calcifications and Cystic Lesions

Placental calcifications are found in over half of pregnancies in the third trimester. Although this can be a normal finding, mothers that use tobacco products, heparin or aspirin therapy secondary to coagulation disorders, and mothers that have delivered fewer babies are more likely to have greater degrees of calcification. Common areas to image placental calcifications are at the septa, base, and around the chorionic and villous spaces. Cystic lesions may also be viewed on sonographic evaluation as a hypoechoic area almost anywhere on the placenta. They are common and usually insignificant.

Placenta Accreta

Placenta accreta describes a condition in which the placenta is abnormally bound to the superficial uterine wall via its villi. If the placental villi penetrate deeper into the uterine muscle layer, the condition is termed placenta accreta. Placenta percreta is the most extreme form placenta accreta, as penetration of the placental villi extends through the entire thickness of the uterus and may even reach surrounding organ structures. The occurrence of placenta accreta is highly correlated with placenta previa. Furthermore, previous cesarean section(s) increases the risk for developing placenta accreta. The primary complication for the baby, in the presence of placenta accreta, is premature delivery. The risk of maternal hemorrhage is the greatest complication of placenta accreta. The abnormally strong and deep attachment of the placenta to the uterus makes placental delivery difficult without tearing and ensuing bleeding of uterine and other structures. An emergent hysterectomy may be indicated.

Placenta accreta should be suspected in any gravid female with placenta previa and an elevated serum alpha-fetoprotein. These findings should be further evaluated with sonography and sometimes MRI. Although definitive prelabor diagnosis is rare, there are characteristic sonographic findings that make the diagnosis more likely. If the muscular area behind the placenta is thinned to less than 2 mm on sonographic measurements, placenta accreta is likely. Irregular, "punched-out" areas of the placenta appearing alternately hypoechoic and anechoic are consistent sonographic findings of placenta accreta. Doppler studies can further accentuate these hypoechoic areas secondary to the rapid blood flow within them.

Battledore Placenta, Velamentous Insertion, and Vasa Previa

All three terms describe abnormal umbilical cord insertion upon the placenta.

- Battledore placenta – a condition in which the umbilical cord inserts on the edge of the placenta rather than its normal central insertion site. This is usually clinically insignificant.
- Velamentous insertion – a condition in which the vessels of the umbilical cord separate and then insert into the edge of the placenta. The separation of the vessels leaves them without the protective gelatinous material. A velamentous insertion increases fetal abnormalities and complications, growth restriction, and preterm labor.
- Vasa previa – a condition in which the vessels of the umbilical cord separate, cross the cervical os and then attach to the edge of the placenta. Vasa previa occurs approximately once every 3,000 births and has a fetal mortality rate of at least 75%.

Circummarginate and Circumvallate

Both conditions affect the normal placental shape. The normal placenta is a discoid shape with membranous edges extending smoothly to the placental edges. Furthermore, the placenta attaches to the uterine wall. Conditions affecting the placental margin result in abnormal placental shape. A circummarginate placenta is a condition in which the fetal chorionic membrane does not reach to the edges of the placenta, from the center. In this situation, the edges of the placenta are covered with a smooth layer of chorion. Similarly, circumvallate placenta is an abnormality in which the fetal chorionic membrane is larger than the placenta and forms folds and prevents a smooth placental edge. Circumvallate placenta can be partial or complete; therefore, it is important to image the entire margin of the placenta. Complete circumvallate placenta is associated with fetal and labor problems. Partial circumvallate placenta and circummarginate placenta are generally not associated with fetal abnormality.

Membranacea and Succenturiate

Both placenta membranacea and placenta succenturiate are conditions that affect normal placental shape. Placenta membranacea is a condition in which the villus of the gestational sac does not regress as through pregnancy. This results in the surface of the gestational sac being entirely covered by placenta. In this condition, the placental membrane will appear abnormally thin. A succenturiate placenta, also known as an accessory lobe, may form in the case of partial placenta membranacea. This accessory placental lobe forms with spotty regression of the villi. The succenturiate is attached to the primary placenta via uterine wall vessels. A succenturiate placental lobe may result in delivery complications.

Accessory Lobe of the Placenta

It is important for ultrasound operators to assess the size and shape of the placenta because it is the lifeline for the fetus. An accessory lobe (succenturiate) is a mass of placental tissue that is connected to the main portion of the placenta by blood vessels. It is important to diagnose an accessory lobe because this area of the placenta may not be delivered with the main lobe of the placenta, and it could cause maternal bleeding after childbirth. Vasa previa is one of the main concerns for the correct identification of an accessory lobe because the vessels may be positioned between the cervix and the presenting fetal anatomy. This may lead to constriction of the blood vessels or rupture of the tissues. If vasa previa is diagnosed, a cesarean section is planned for the patient. An accessory lobe of the placenta is found about 5% of the time.

Ultrasound Appearance

The placenta is a curved organ that attaches to the uterine wall during pregnancy. This organ supplies the fetus with oxygen and nutrients, and it clears wastes from the fetal circulation. The placenta is disk shaped, extremely vascular, and separated into maternal and fetal divisions. When a patient has an accessory lobe of the placenta, it can be classified as one of three types including succenturiate, bipartite, and annular placentas. A succenturiate lobe will be identified by ultrasound as an additional (yet smaller) component of the placenta that is connected to the main portion by blood vessels. A bipartite placenta (also referred to as a bilobed placenta) appears as two placental lobes also connected by blood vessels. As opposed to the succenturiate lobe, these divisions of the placenta are the same size and are connected by chorionic tissue that provides a thin connection of the two lobes. An annular placenta is one that forms a ring around the internal uterus. All of these are important to document so that placental retention does not create bleeding or infection after the child is born.

Amniotic Band Syndrome

Amniotic band syndrome is a condition in which many congenital malformations are present ranging from mild to complex. An example of a mild malformation is lymphedema of the digits due to constriction bands. An example of complex defects from amniotic band syndrome is fetal limb amputation. The constricting bands of tissue seen in this syndrome can affect almost any part of the fetal anatomy. Ambiguous genitalia, facial clefts and severe abdominal wall deformities are also seen in amniotic band syndrome. The prevalence of amniotic band syndrome is approximately 7 in every 10,000 live births. Amniotic band syndrome should be differentiated from body stalk anomalies and the presence of an amniotic sheet, versus constricting amniotic bands, when performing the sonogram.

Chorioangioma

A chorioangioma is a benign vascular tumor of the placenta. As its name would suggest, it arises from chorionic tissue. Determining whether a chorioangioma is at high-risk for causing fetal or maternal difficulties is dependent on two variables: size and vascularity. Any chorioangioma greater than 5 cm increases the risk for complications. The greater blood flow (determined with Doppler studies), the more likely fetal complications will develop. Sonographically, a chorioangioma is usually visualized at the insertion site of the placental cord. It will appear as a clearly demarcated and round lesion. Careful evaluation of the fetus for conditions of volume overload and hydrops is necessary in the event of visualizing a chorioangioma. Regular sonographic monitoring is indicated.

Vascular Umbilical Cord Abnormalities

The most common (1% of pregnancies) vascular abnormality of the umbilical cord is the presence of only one umbilical artery instead of two. This should be evaluated at the fetal end of the umbilical cord, not the placental end, to avoid arterial fusion, which is a normal variant. The absence of the second umbilical artery is likely from clotting in the artery, resulting in infarction. If a single umbilical cord artery is confirmed, about a 40% chance of other fetal abnormalities and malformation exists. Rarely, an increased number of umbilical cord vessels may be noted. This condition is known as a multivessel cord and is associated with conjoined twins and fetal malformation.

Abnormal Umbilical Cord

Short Umbilical Cord

Abnormal embryologic development and folding of cord material usually starts at about the 4th to 5th week of development. The same conditions that result in complete lack of umbilical cord formation can also result in short cord syndrome. Sometimes an umbilical cord can form from fetal abdominal wall material (body stalk anomaly). A short umbilical cord restricts fetal movement resulting in a number of fetal abnormalities including: cord compression, placental abruption, limb abnormalities, body wall defects, fetal heart rate abnormalities and compromised fetal descent during labor. Insufficient amniotic fluid, multiple pregnancy, maternal use of cocaine, amniotic bands, and other fetal abnormalities correlate with the finding of short umbilical cord.

Long Umbilical Cord

The term long cord is often synonymous with nuchal cord or nuchal loops. Nuchal loops may be found in up to 25% of pregnancies. Nuchal cords are a condition in which the umbilical cord is looped (at least twice) around the fetal neck. An abnormally long umbilical cord is more likely to be associated with cord knots and cord prolapse. Umbilical cord prolapse is seen in up to 1 in 300 pregnancies. A prolapse occurs when a portion or loop of umbilical cord slips into the vaginal canal after membranes rupture but before the baby descends into the birth canal. All of the above aforementioned conditions can still result in a healthy baby, but there may be a higher incidence of fetal heart rate patterns, amniotic meconium, and cesarean delivery. Nuchal cord and long cord abnormalities present complications because of the stretching and/or compression they place on umbilical cord vessels.

Umbilical Cord Masses

Umbilical cord hemangiomas are often seen near the placental end of the cord as an echogenic area. Edema may be visualized beyond the actual area of hemangioma. This may involve bleeding, fetal anemia and hydrops. A cord hemangioma can be differentiated by an umbilical cord teratoma by the presence of sonographic calcifications within the echogenic cord mass. An aneurysm is another cord mass that may be sonographically visualized as a local dilation of any of the umbilical vessels. These can clot and cause fetal death. An umbilical cord hematoma occurs in approximately 1 in every 500 births. Increasing incidence is secondary to increased amniocentesis and cord blood sampling. This can usually be seen near the fetal end of the umbilical cord and is usually the result of the fetal umbilical vein being ruptured. Fetal mortality is variable but as high as 50%.

Umbilical Cord Cysts

Three main types of umbilical cord cysts exist. If cysts are visualized in the first trimester, they may resolve or turn out to be a normal variant. Second and third trimester cysts may be associated with increased concern for fetal anomalies. The first type is omphalomesenteric duct cyst. This cyst arises from yolk stalk tissue and is viewed with ultrasound near the fetal end of the umbilical cord insertion. The second type of umbilical cord cyst is the allantois or urachus duct cyst. Embryologically, this structure extends from the fetal bladder to the umbilical cord. This type of cyst is often seen near the fetal end, separates the umbilical vessels, and is associated with fetal abnormalities. Thirdly, a pseudocyst is from inflammation of the Wharton's jelly. The umbilical vessels can travel through these cysts and the cysts are usually insignificant and sometimes resolve on their own.

Abnormal Umbilical Cord Structural Formation

The presence of a structurally abnormal or absent umbilical cord usually has a fatal prognosis for the fetus. Structural cord abnormalities are secondary to an abnormal embryonic folding that results in fetal abdominal wall malformation. Without an umbilical cord, the fetus is directly attached to the placenta. On sonographic evaluation the umbilical cord will not be visualized and the fetal abdominal organs will appear herniated or outside of the fetal body. Limb abnormalities may also be visualized. This condition is also termed: congenital absence/aplasia of the umbilical cord, body stalk anomaly, or limb-body wall complex.

Cervix and Maternal Pathology

Cervical Incompetence

Shortening

Cervical incompetence is a rare complication of pregnancy but could be the cause of a miscarriage in the second trimester. In the pregnant population, ultrasound is the preferred imaging modality to examine the cervix. A transvaginal approach is favored in cases of suspected cervical incompetence. Otherwise, this can be assessed transabdominally during the second-trimester anatomy scan. In this case, if the cervix measures less than 35 mm, the sonographer should measure it again with a transvaginal approach. During a transvaginal exam, the operator should have the patient void the bladder prior to the exam. Obtain a long-axis view of the cervix, and measure the cervical canal from the internal os to the external os. It is recommended to repeat this three times and use the shortest measurement. The sonographer should observe the cervix for at least five minutes to determine if there is funneling. A cervix that measures less than 25 mm is concerning if there have been previous pregnancy losses or if this is detected before 24 weeks of gestation. Some facilities will also require a cervical stress test in which fundal pressure is applied for 15 seconds and the cervix is measured another three times.

Funneling

Cervical incompetence may be responsible for a premature birth or even the loss of a pregnancy in the second trimester. Sonographers will check the cervical length along with any evidence of funneling. Funneling occurs when the amniotic sac extends into the cervix. Sonographers should observe the cervix for at least five minutes to note any changes. Often, if funneling is noted, the cervix will be shortened (less than 25 mm) so the cervical length should also be recorded. Most facilities do not require a measurement of the cervical width and depth, but it is important to document the absence or presence of funneling so it can be reported.

Cerclage

Cervical incompetence is a risk for women with congenital uterine defects, repeated procedures that required dilation of the cervix, and cone biopsies. Women with cervical incompetence experience a preterm birth or pregnancy loss in the second trimester. Management for women who are at risk for preterm delivery due to cervical incompetence may include bed rest, pharmaceuticals, or a procedure called cervical cerclage. A cervical cerclage may be performed in an emergency or for those that have already suffered a previous miscarriage or premature baby. If performed to safeguard the pregnancy, this is often done between 12 and 15 weeks of gestation. During this procedure, the physician will place a suture around the cervix so it remains closed. Often, this stitch is removed around 37 weeks of gestation. These sutures can be visualized sonographically within the middle portion of the cervix.

Maternal Hypertension

Hypertension in pregnancy is defined similarly as that of a non-pregnant person as a blood pressure higher than 140/90. It can also be defined as an increase in blood pressure higher than 30/15 as compared to average pre-pregnancy measurements. Furthermore, abnormal blood pressure recordings must be obtained on two separate occasions at least 6 hours apart to diagnose maternal hypertension. Maternal hypertension usually develops in the third trimester in up to 10% of pregnancies that proceed to this stage. The risk increases substantially in a multiple gestation. Maternal hypertension carries increased risks of morbidity and mortality for both the mother and fetus.

The two most common pregnancy-induced hypertensive disorders are preeclampsia and eclampsia. Preeclampsia is defined as the development of the triad of hypertension, proteinuria, and edema during pregnancy. This is further subdivided into mild and severe depending on the degrees of the three conditions. Preeclampsia usually develops around the second half of pregnancy. Eclampsia is defined when all of the criteria for preeclampsia are met plus the presence of convulsions. Eclampsia is more commonly seen in the first 72 postpartum hours. Sonographic findings of intrauterine growth restriction, decreased placental volume or rapid placental maturation, insufficient amniotic fluid amounts, and fetal demise are correlated with a preeclamptic pregnancy. Doppler studies may show vascular resistance in the placenta.

Preterm Labor

Preterm labor is defined as regular contractions, cervical dilation, and ruptured membranes prior to gestational week 37. Approximately 12% of births are premature and of these, 25% are intentional or induced preterm labor for medical reasons. About 75% of preterm labors are spontaneous. Risk factors for preterm labor include maternal infection, smoking, drug/alcohol use, poor nutrition, and stress. Maternal infections, chronic maternal disease states and maternal socioeconomic status have also been implicated. Preterm labor is more likely with multiple gestation, placental abnormalities, maternal anatomical anomalies, and fetal abnormalities. Assessment of preterm labor includes evaluation of the maternal cervix and cervical secretions looking for the presence of a protein fibronectin. Monitoring of force and frequency of uterine contractions with a tocodynamometer may be used (less frequently) to assess risk of preterm labor. Sonographic assessment of preterm labor by measurement of cervical length measurement is a commonly used diagnostic tool as well.

Pelvic Masses

Many gynecological conditions may exist prior to a woman becoming gravid. These conditions may or may not have been symptomatic in the pregravidic state. Pregnancy may result in these preexisting conditions becoming noticeable or identified if they were previously asymptomatic. On the other hand, if symptoms did exist prior to conception, they may intensify during pregnancy. Sonographically speaking, gynecological conditions can be broken down into 2 categories: the presence of a palpable and sonographically identifiable pelvic mass and areas of referred pain that can be evaluated sonographically (flank, abdomen, and extremities). Sonographic masses less than 5 cm of non-obstetrical origin may be monitored with the watch and wait approach. Surgical consideration must be given to all other masses. The primary limiting factor in detecting pelvic masses is maternal obesity.

A corpus luteum cyst is the most common occurring ovarian mass seen in pregnancy. They are generally small, but can reach a size greater than 5 cm. Regardless of the size, a large percentage of corpus luteum cysts resolve by the 18th gestational week. In the case of a corpus luteum cyst that is greater than 5 cm and symptomatic (pelvic or abdominal pain), surgical intervention may be considered due to the increased risk of bleeding into itself and twisting on itself (torsion). Higher incidences of these cysts are seen in females that have used fertility drugs such as Clomid.

Hydrosalpinx and Cystadenoma

Hydrosalpinx is a fluid collection in one or both fallopian tubes that may become obstructing. It may occur as the result of a pelvic infection. The history of this in a pregravidic female may raise fertility concerns. Found during obstetrical ultrasound, it may be visualized as a rounded cyst with multiple septations. Hydrosalpinx must be differentiated from a cystadenoma. A cystadenoma is the most common cystic ovarian tumor. The sonographic appearance varies greatly, from a cystic mass without septations to a cystic mass with multiple thin or thick septations. The sonographic appearance of nodules in a cystadenoma increases the concern for malignancy.

Solid Pelvic Masses

In the presence of a sonographic finding of a solid mass during obstetrical sonography, it is important to determine whether this mass arises from the ovary or the uterus. In the presence of the sonographic "claw sign" (uterine distortion around the solid mass), the solid mass arises from the uterus. In the absence of uterine distortion, the solid mass likely originates from the ovary. Masses associated with pregnancy include: leiomyomas, uterine fibroids, solid ovarian masses, and focal myometrial contraction. Leiomyomas are the most common and sonographically appear with a well-defined border and usually hyperechoic; in some instances, they may contain central cysts. Documentation of mass location and growth is important in prenatal planning and monitoring, as solid masses can affect placental implantation and delivery.

Dermoid Cysts and Pelvic Kidney

The sonographic finding of a dermoid cyst during pregnancy presents as an echogenic and complex mass with posterior shadowing. Within the mass are the appearance of ectodermal structures such as hair, skin and teeth. Definitive and recommended treatment is removal. A pelvic maternal kidney may be an incidental sonographic finding during pregnancy. Sonographically it is viewed as either a complex or sold mass and may contain cysts located centrally within the mass. The presence of hydronephrosis is the greatest concern during pregnancy.

Non-Gynecologic Maternal Disorders

Several non-gynecological maternal disorders causing pain may coexist with a normal pregnancy. We will limit this discussion to disorders that have an increased propensity to develop during pregnancy and those that can be successfully evaluated and diagnosed with sonography. Acute cholecystitis may occur as the result of preexisting gallstones or the development of stones during pregnancy. Appendicitis may occur during pregnancy. Sonographically, look for the appendix to be more superior and laterally located (in the gravid patient) to its normal anatomical position. Pyelonephritis may be sonographically evaluated in the presence of localized flank pain and a positive urine culture. Deep vein thrombosis can best be diagnosed with venous duplex ultrasound. Ureteral calculus may occur and may be diagnosed with sonography and/or intravenous urogram to assess obstruction.

Maternal Alloimmunization

Maternal alloimmunization or isoimmunization is also known as Rh incompatibility. This occurs when a mother has rhesus or Rh-negative blood and her fetus has Rh-positive blood. When the mother's Rh-negative blood comes into contact with the fetus Rh-positive blood cells, through placental nourishment, the mother makes antibodies against the Rh-positive blood cells. These antibodies against the Rh-positive blood may cross the placenta and start to destroy fetal red blood cells. The first pregnancy is usually not affected, but successive pregnancies may be affected and Rh incompatibility can cause a range of problems for the fetus, from mild to fatal. Hemolysis can occur, resulting in a jaundiced baby. Severe and even fatal fetal complications of Rh incompatibility are hydrops fetalis and kernicterus.

TORCH Infections

TORCH infections are a group of five common intrauterine infections that physicians and sonographers should be aware of during the reproductive years of a woman's life. TORCH is an acronym for toxoplasmosis, other, rubella, cytomegalovirus, and herpes simplex virus (types 1 and 2). Providers can test for TORCH, but this may first be diagnosed during an abnormal OB ultrasound. When the fetus is affected, physicians can provide more thorough and effective prenatal and antenatal care for the fetus as well as provide better care in any subsequent pregnancies. Ultrasound indicators of TORCH include intrauterine growth restriction, microcephaly, hydrocephalus, calcifications within the brain, cataracts, cardiac malformations, and fetal hydrops. If mothers have not been tested for these infections, they may not be aware of the risk associated with passing these infections onto their babies. Not all babies with TORCH can be diagnosed sonographically because sometimes the infections cause intellectual disabilities and sensory issues.

Protocols and Procedures

Clinical Standards and Guidelines

Importance of Correlating Findings from Previous Ultrasound Exams

Often, pelvic and OB ultrasound exams are performed in order to follow up on pathology or to track the well-being and progression of the fetus. If a follow-up scan of an ovarian cyst or uterine fibroid is requested, it is important that the sonographer examines the prior ultrasound and report in order to know the number, size, and location of these structures. Today's ultrasound systems allow the sonographer to import parameters from previous OB studies in order to track interval growth of a fetus. Graphs can be used by the clinicians to serve as a visual aid in understanding the growth that has taken place. It is also important to compare previous studies because clinicians should not redact the estimated date of delivery if an exam was performed correctly earlier in the pregnancy. Follow-up scans for interval growth should not be performed weekly because the measurements may be incorrectly evaluated because a margin of error can exist. It is typically suggested that these follow-up exams are performed over a span that ranges from two to four weeks.

Fusion Imaging

Fusion imaging (also known as hybrid imaging) is a technique that provides sonographers and clinicians with greater diagnostic confidence when following up lesions discovered on previous computed tomography (CT) or magnetic resonance imaging (MRI) studies. Fusion imaging also reduces the amount of radiation that a patient is exposed to because ultrasound does not use radiation. Still another advantage is greater dynamic monitoring during invasive procedures. Real-time virtual sonography is one example of hybrid imaging that allows gray-scale, color Doppler, or the use of contrast harmonics and CT or MRI images to be displayed simultaneously. The CT or MRI images must be sent to the ultrasound system so that the same cross-sectional image can be recreated with sonography. Fusion imaging requires a sensor that is attached to the transducer that determines the probe location during the scan as well as a transmitter that is attached to the patient.so the sonographer knows the suspicious lesion is being evaluated.

Acetylcholinesterase

Acetylcholinesterase (ACHE) is a protein that can be evaluated during pregnancy to determine increased risks for the development of neural tube defects in a fetus. The test is usually only used after a positive AFP test. ACHE testing is done via amniocentesis. Although ACHE testing offers greater specificity for fetal neurological defect determination, it may also be positive in a number of other fetal abnormalities. It should be used in conjunction with other maternal screening tests and not independently. The triple maternal screen incorporates testing of AFP, unconjugated estriol, and human chorionic gonadotropin to determine risk for fetal chromosomal anomalies. Maternal triple screening specifically evaluates the risk of delivering a baby with Down syndrome and trisomy 18. False positive rates for the triple screen are as high as 6%.

Alpha-Fetoprotein Testing

Alpha-fetoprotein (AFP) testing of the maternal serum is ideally performed at about 14-16 weeks gestation. This level measures the amount of the protein in maternal circulation. Alpha-fetoprotein is produced by the fetal liver and the yolk sac in all pregnancies. The AFP increases throughout a pregnancy until the 32nd week. For the AFP testing to be optimal, an accurate gestational age must be present. The maternal serum AFP level for gestational age must be within 2 multiples of the median, which is taken from a population of same-gestational-age women. Therefore, AFP testing is partly a biological and partly a statistical test. Higher-than-expected maternal serum levels suggest increase likelihood of fetal neural tube or abdominal wall defects. Lower-than-expected maternal serum AFP levels suggest increased likelihood of chromosomal anomalies such as Down syndrome.

Pelvic Preparation for Sonography

As with any patient encounter, a brief introduction and a thorough history are imperative. Do not rely solely on the sonography order, as this may contain human error or if handwritten, penmanship may be difficult to read. Question the patient about their symptoms and their location, allergies, past surgeries, and what exam they are having done. Not only does this support the order for the imaging study, but gives you a clue as to the patients experience with such a procedure. Determining if previous imaging studies have been done on the pelvis/abdomen, as well as dates and location is helpful for comparison and interpretation. The procedure should be explained and questions and concerns answered. Equipment should be properly cleaned, and protocols followed. It is often recommended that the transducer sheath or condom be placed over the transducer while the patient is observing, further reassuring the patient of infectious disease control.

Sonography

Transabdominal sonographs are commonly used to evaluate pelvic structures and organs. This technique is especially useful in evaluation of upper uterine and pelvic masses, ovaries and ectopic pregnancies. It is also widely used in the gravid female, for fetal monitoring and assessment. Transabdominal sonography may be synonymous with pelvic sonography. It may be done with a full urinary bladder to enhance the appearance of some structures. An endovaginal or transvaginal sonography allows for view of pelvic structures, especially those that are more inferiorly and posteriorly located. These sonographs are usually of greater quality. It is important for the technician to thoroughly describe this procedure to the patient prior to introducing the vaginal probe. Sonohysterography is used primarily to evaluate the endometrial structures, as a catheter is introduced into the endometrium, filling it with sterile saline solution.

Endovaginal Sonography

Transabdominal or pelvic sonography is a useful and well-tolerated procedure indicated for a number of conditions. Irregular vaginal bleeding, dyspareunia, pelvic pain, and signs of pelvic infection may require pelvic ultrasound as part of the diagnostic work-up. It is used to evaluate any pelvic mass and is just as often used to "rule-out" ectopic pregnancy as to diagnose it. It is also used to monitor and assess fetal growth. Endovaginal or transvaginal sonography is contraindicated in the patient with an intact hymen, virgin patient, and premenarchal patient. Furthermore, this test may be refused by any number of patients, for a multitude of reasons including religious beliefs. Endovaginal ultrasound is not indicated for those patients that have received endovaginal radiation treatments.

Translabial Ultrasound

A translabial (also referred to as transperineal) ultrasound exam can be performed with a 4–8 MHz transducer (curved array) or by using the endovaginal transducer if penetration of the ultrasound beam is not required. A protective cover is placed over the probe face. Gel is applied in the cover as well as on the external surface in order to conduct the sound waves.

The patient should be in the lithotomy position on an exam table used for pelvic scans, or a cushion should be used to elevate the hips. The operator should start in a sagittal orientation to identify the cervix and use the bladder as a landmark. The vagina will be positioned between the urinary bladder and the rectum. The probe may need to be rotated to help get rid of gas or to avoid shadowing from the pubic bone.

Translabial Method

Sometimes, the more conventional methods of performing an ultrasound are contraindicated or additional views are required to provide clinicians with a correct diagnosis. The translabial technique may be beneficial during a pelvic, OB, or bladder ultrasound. A translabial (also referred to as transperineal) approach can be performed when an endovaginal ultrasound exam cannot be performed or if it is too painful for the patient. A translabial approach is a useful method to measure the cervix or assess the placenta and lower genitourinary structures in cases of placenta previa. This is the ultrasound method of choice in cases of uterine prolapse or incontinence. The translabial method can add value because imaging with this technique can also be done in multiple planes. The ultrasound user should always be familiar with anatomy when performing additional views.

Detection of Torsion

Torsion refers to the twisting along the long axis of an adnexal mass or cyst, thus compromising blood supply. Torsion is always accompanied by a maternal complaint of pain, usually pelvic. Torsion can be very difficult to diagnose; therefore, whenever there is a maternal complaint of pain, one must maintain an increased index of suspicion for torsion. Furthermore, the diagnosis is broken into partial and complete torsion. Doppler evaluation is ideal but not always absolutely diagnostic due to varied blood flow to ovaries under normal circumstances. Sonography is most accurate when there is a small mass; torsion is then more obvious as the affected ovary becomes edematous, enlarged, and with multiple cysts.

Paraovarian Cysts

A paraovarian cyst is sonographically differentiated from an ovarian cyst by its location outside of the ovary. It is located within the broad ligament and arises as a result of the embryonic remnants of the Wolffian ducts. It is rarely symptomatic and therefore is usually an incidental sonographic finding. Its sonographic appearance is a rounded cyst with septae located adjacent to the ovary. Although usually asymptomatic, paraovarian cysts are noteworthy because of their risk of torsion. Risk of torsion is greater in the pregnant versus the nonpregnant patient.

Measurement Techniques

Protocols for Adnexa Evaluation

The American Institute of Ultrasound in Medicine (AIUM) has established examination and documentation protocols for evaluation of the adnexa. The ovaries are the primary structure that should be identified and thoroughly described in sonography of the adnexa. The ovaries should serve as the primary landmark in sonographic examination of the adnexa. In the case of an enlarged uterus or a postmenopausal patient, the ovaries may not be readily imaged; in every other instance, every attempt should be made to document visualization of the ovaries. It is important to document size and thickness in all planes, location, and the presence of any masses and their description and measurements. Compare all findings to the opposite ovary. The fallopian tubes need to be part of the adnexal sonography and description. However, in the absence of pathology, fallopian tubes are generally not identified on sonography. Any fallopian tube visualization should contain all appropriate descriptors, measurements and notes on symmetry.

Sonographic Uterus Evaluation

Sonographic evaluation of the uterus is not only important to diagnose uterine-related disorders, but often equally important as a reference point to evaluating other structures within the pelvic cavity. Thorough documentation of this structure is imperative; particularly uterine size (in all planes), uterine shape and position, endometrial lining (thickness and both layers and all planes), myometrial lining (thickness and description), and cervical appearance (size, orientation, mass). If there is fluid present within any of these structures, do not include it in the measurement itself; rather, fluid gets its own description and measurement.

Crown-Rump Length

Once the embryo can be visualized with ultrasound, the crown-rump length measurement becomes the most accurate and preferred method of gestational age determination. In this situation, the gestational sac diameter measurements are no longer useful for gestational age determination. The embryo can me visualized when it is as small as 2 mm; this often correlates with a gestational age of about 6 weeks. The most accurate crown-rump length, and thus most accurate gestational age, should be taken from the average of three good measurements at maximal length. Although the embryo can be imaged earlier, a clearer sonographic image is established after week seven.

Measuring the Yolk Sac

The yolk sac is often the first structure visualized within the gestational sac during an early pregnancy because it can be identified even earlier than the embryonic pole. When an extremely early intrauterine pregnancy is identified sonographically, the yolk sac may be the only structure visible (other than the gestational sac). The yolk sac can be measured to provide clinicians with information about the pregnancy or when the yolk sac appears abnormal (shape, size, solidity, or calcification). Measurements should be taken from the inner leading edge to the opposite inner leading edge. Yolk sacs that measure greater than 6 mm without the presence of a fetal pole suggest fetal demise, and this should be followed up accordingly. Ultrasound users should be aware that the number of yolk sacs will be the same as the number of amniotic sacs as long as the embryos are alive.

The yolk sac is an important structure to evaluate with ultrasound in the first trimester of pregnancy. The yolk sac provides the embryo with nutrients until the placenta is fully developed and provides the required nourishment. In a very early pregnancy, the yolk sac is one of the first extraembryonic structures that can be identified during an OB ultrasound. First, the gestational sac will be visualized with the yolk sac becoming visible during week 5 before an embryonic pole can be identified. It is important that the operator look at the sonographic characteristics of the yolk sac as well as the size. Yolk sacs should not have an irregular shape (the typical appearance is round), and they should not be calcified or resemble a solid mass. These characteristics can be a good indicator of the well-being of the fetus.

Nuchal Translucency

Nuchal translucency measurements deserve much attention. Accurate sonographic measurement is highly technique and position dependent. Misinterpretation or measurement can result in a misinformed patient and mismanaged pregnancy. The nuchal translucency test measures the hypoechoic space between the back of the fetal neck and the skin overlying this area. However, it is an "inside to inside" measurement that should only measure the translucent portions and not the skin or soft tissue. It is best measured with the fetus neck flexed. If possible, observe fetal movement away from the amniotic sac periphery, so that unfused amnion is not mistaken with fetal skin for accurate measurement end points. It is first visible on sonograph at 10 weeks. At about 14 weeks, nuchal translucency measurements are maximal up to 2.8 mm, and then thins through the rest of the pregnancy. Both transabdominal and endovaginal measurements are recommended.

Biparietal Measurements

Sonographic biparietal diameter measurements are best obtained at about week 14. To obtain the most accurate measurements, the following three anatomical structures must be clearly identifiable: the midline falx, symmetrical thalami, and the cavum septum pellucidum. A high degree of accuracy can still be obtained with measurements through any plane that crosses through the thalami and ventricle. This forms an oval shape and measurements should be recorded from leading edges at greatest width of the oval. The transducer must remain perpendicular to the parietal bones during measurements. Limitations for accurate sonographic biparietal diameter measurements include later gestational age, increased transducer pressure on the abdomen, abnormal fetal position, and a fetus with a "flat head". In these instances, use measurements in conjunction with head circumference, cephalic index and femur length to determine the most accurate gestational age.

The biparietal diameter (BPD) is one of the main measurements used to determine fetal weight and gestational age. This measurement is typically performed in the second trimester; the CRL is often used in the first trimester. The BPD can be measured at the widest level that includes the third ventricle, thalami, and cavum septum pellucidum. The first cursor should be placed on the outer edge of the skull closest to the transducer with the second set at the inner edge of the skull that is farthest away from the probe. One main disadvantage of using the BPD is that it is affected by the shape of the skull. When BPD shape correction is used, the BPD will be the same as the head circumference (HC). The accuracy of the HC is not affected by the shape of the head. The following formula can be used for the shape-corrected BPD, where OFD is the occipitofrontal diameter:

$$\text{shape corrected BPD} = \text{BPD} \times \frac{\text{OFD}}{1.265}$$

Measuring Head Circumference

Measurement of fetal head circumference is useful in determining fetal age and making fetal weight determinations. Fetal head circumference measurements are essentially an average of two measurements: the biparietal diameter and the anterior/posterior diameter. Therefore, many of the landmarks used to measure biparietal diameter, need also be located for head circumference measurements. Measurements should be taken through the third ventricle and thalamus. The posterior brain should contain visualization of the tentorial hiatus and the anterior brain should show the cavum septum pellucidi. Sonographic measurement arrows should be placed on the outer calvarial wall edges opposite each other, but should not contain the outer skin edge.

Fetal head circumference measurements should be taken with the transducer positioned correctly from three planes. Optimal fetal head circumference measurements will be obtained when the plane is parallel to that of the skull base. This arranges the plane in the anterior portion of the cranium. This plane may also be known as the transverse axial plane. A measurement perpendicular to the above aforementioned plane should also be taken, from outer edge to outer edge; this is known as the occipitofrontal or anterior/posterior diameter measurement.

Measuring the Cerebellum

The cerebellum is a dumbbell-shaped structure in the posterior fossa that is situated just anterior to the cisterna magna. Abnormal measurements of these posterior fossa structures can provide clinicians with clues about Dandy–Walker malformation. One such example that a sonographer should look for is the simultaneous visualization of an enlarged cisterna magna and a malformation of the cerebellar vermis that provides a pathway between the cisterna magna and the fourth ventricle. To measure the cerebellum, the calipers should be placed on the outer margins of the cerebellum. The transcerebellar diameter distance has been found to correlate well with the gestational age in weeks (if you drop the period), and it may be useful because this measurement is not dependent on the shape of the head. The transcerebellar diameter measurement can also be helpful in providing another parameter to estimate the age for twins as well.

Importance of Evaluating the Cerebellum

The development of the cerebellum is quite extensive because it is one of the first areas to develop in the brain, but it is one of the last portions of the brain to be formed completely. The cerebellum is one of the main portions of the brain that is essential for motor function such as coordination, performing fine motor movements, and balance. The cerebellum is located in the posterior fossa, and it can be imaged when moving the probe to an inferior and posterior position from where the biparietal diameter and head circumference measurements are taken. The cerebellum will appear as a dumbbell-shaped structure, and transcerebellar diameter measurements can be provided. The cisterna magna will be located posterior to the cerebellum with the nuchal fold just posterior to the bone of the skull.

Importance of Measuring the Cisterna Magna

A thorough evaluation of the posterior fossa will include measurements of the cisterna magna. This anatomic structure receives cerebral spinal fluid from the fourth ventricle of the brain. Normal parameters for the cisterna magna during a 2D ultrasound exam fall between 2- and 10-mm. Mega cisterna magna is suspected for any measurement greater than 10 mm, and if it is determined that the cisterna magna is connected to the fourth ventricle, then Dandy–Walker malformation should be considered. Dandy–Walker malformation may aid in the diagnosis of any chromosomal abnormalities because it has been associated with trisomy 13, 18, and 21. It is important to diagnose these abnormalities as early as possible to help the family decide on the direction of the rest of the pregnancy. Trisomy 18 is a deadly disorder that typically causes spontaneous abortion or causes the baby to be stillborn, and those with trisomy 13 typically die shortly after they are born. Imaging in 3D can also be used to document and measure the cisterna magna.

Binocular and Transcerebellar Measurements

Sonographic binocular measurements and transcerebellar measurements are rarely used in obstetrics to determine gestational age, especially with all of the other options and measurements available and their high degree of accuracy. However, in rare circumstances, binocular and transcerebellar measurements may be used to determine gestational age if fetal head and femur measurements cannot be obtained. Binocular measurements can be obtained with the fetal head in the occipital posterior position. In this position, measure the diameter of the outer orbits to estimate gestational age. With transcerebellar diameter measurements in the transverse direction, then measurement in millimeters should equal that of the gestational week.

Cephalic Index

The cephalic index is useful to obtain accurate sonographic measurements despite variants in fetal head shape. Some head shape variants can be greater, especially in circumstances of breech fetal position, ruptured membranes and multiple gestations. The cephalic index is an equation that divides occipitofrontal measurements into biparietal diameter measurements and multiplies this by 100. It should be noted that a true biparietal diameter is not used in this equation, rather the maximal width, perpendicular to the maximal anterior/posterior length, is used. Expected values are between 74 and 83. A second equation may be used based on an "ideal" cephalic index of 78. This equation takes the total of the multiplied biparietal and occipitofrontal diameters and multiplies it by 1.265. The result is the "shape-corrected biparietal diameter".

Measuring Nuchal Fold, Femur, and Renal Pelvis

Measurements of the nuchal fold, femur, and renal pelvis should be standard and performed whether one is looking for Down syndrome, other anomalies, or evaluating a normal fetus. The nuchal fold is best measured with the fetal head in the transverse plane. Measurement is taken from outer occipital bone to inner skin margin and should be less than 7 mm. Nuchal thickening may resolve later in pregnancy. After obtaining sonographic fetal femur measurements, the following equation should be utilized:

$$0.9028 \times \text{biparietal diameter} - 9.3105 = \text{expected femur length}$$

If there is approximately a 10% reduction in actual and expected femur measurements, suspect Down syndrome. Down syndrome may also be suspected if fetal anteroposterior diameter measurements of the renal pelvis are greater than 3 mm.

Abdominal Circumference

Measurement of fetal abdominal circumference via sonography is the least accurate method of gestational age determination. The decreased accuracy of abdominal circumference measurements is due to several different factors. First, it is difficult in a technical sense, because the abdomen is not symmetrical. Second, landmarks are difficult to locate consistently. Third, the margins are not as clearly defined and visualized on sonography like those of the calvarium of the head. Fourth, excessive transducer pressure can distort the abdominal shape and thus the abdominal circumference measurements. Finally, the abdominal cavity is highly affected by fetal abnormalities and therefore measurements may be quite variable in this circumstance.

For optimal abdominal circumference measurements, location of abdominal landmarks and positioning in the correct plane is necessary. Locate the lower ribs, as these are symmetric and usually readily identifiable. Locate the liver (the largest fetal abdominal organ) and the point at which its length is greatest from end to end. The greatest 'diameter' of the liver is usually found where the left and right portal veins become continuous with each other. The optimal plane for this is the cephalocaudal plane. In this plane, be sure the umbilical segment of the left portal vein is at its shortest. Measurements are from skin edge to skin edge; do not mistake these for the rib edges. Add the transverse diameter plus the anteroposterior diameter and multiply by 1.57 to obtain abdominal circumference.

The "round rule" may be utilized with sonographic measurements of abdominal circumference when less than optimal circumstances present themselves. The most common of these situations would be difficulty locating the fetal landmarks required for abdominal circumference measurements. If this is the case, measure the anteroposterior diameter and transverse diameter where they are thought to be approximately equal. Abdominal circumference measurement results when using the "round rule" will not be highly accurate but they will be acceptable as long as care is taken to not apply too great of transducer pressure.

Length of the Humerus

When an OB ultrasound is performed between 18 and 22 weeks, most of the bones of the extremities will be able to be identified. The humerus length (HL) is a common long bone measurement that is used in addition to the femur length to estimate gestational age and weight. It is important to note that when measuring the HL, the operator should make every attempt to make sure that it is laid out in a horizontal orientation on the monitor with the more superficial limb being measured. This will enable the sonographer to visualize the entire diaphysis of the bone and reduce any possible errors associated with foreshortening. The calipers should be placed at the areas that are the most reflective at the proximal and distal ends of the humerus, taking care not to include the epiphyseal end of the bone. If the humerus tends to be shorter, several measurements should be taken, and skeletal dysplasia should be considered.

Fetal Femur Length

Sonographic measurement of the fetal femur length is less important as a gestational age determinant than it is to determine fetal skeletal growth and exclude anomalies such as dwarfism. Sonographic technique should begin with the transducer positioned at abdominal circumference. The transducer should then be moved in the inferior direction, transecting the bladder. At this position, the transducer should be rotated about 30 degrees for optimal femur viewing. If the angle is greater than 30 degrees to the horizontal, femur length measurements will not be accurate. Furthermore, measurements are only accurate if taken from two blunted ends. The femoral head and greater trochanter are not included in the measurement. Do not mistake the tibia for the femur and remember the femur is straight on the lateral side and curved on the medial side.

Other Bones Measured During an OB Ultrasound

It may be necessary to measure the long bones of the forearm and lower leg to provide additional information pertaining to abnormalities of the appendicular skeleton. As with the femur and humerus, only the ossified portion of the bone should be measured when the bone is in a horizontal orientation on the screen. The bones of the forearm include the radius (positioned on the thumb side) and ulna (located on the side of the fifth digit). The ulna is longer than the radius because it articulates with the humerus in the elbow joint. If the hand is pronated, the sonographer should be aware that the two bones will appear to be situated on top of one another. In the lower leg, the operator should demonstrate two bones of almost equal length with the tibia being the bone positioned medially and the fibula laterally. The operator should take a picture of the foot positioned perpendicular to the lower leg.

BIOPHYSICAL PROFILE

The biophysical profile is one of several methods used to assess fetal well-being. The biophysical profile grades five areas of well-being, giving each category a score of "0" for abnormal or a score of "2" for normal. The five areas evaluated are: fetal breathing movements, fetal body movement, fetal tone, reactive fetal heart rate (nonstress test), and amniotic fluid volume. The scores are added together and a score of 8-10 indicates normal fetal well-being. A score of 6 is equivocal and a score of less than or equal to 4 is abnormal.

SIGNS OF FETAL DISTRESS

In terms of biophysical profile markers, acute fetal distress can be diagnosed with a score of "0" in any of the categories. Fetal distress is present if there are no fetal breath movements for 30 consecutive seconds in a 30-minute monitoring period. Acute fetal distress may be present if there are less than 3 fetal body/limb movements in 30 minutes. Fetal tone assessment that reveals a flaccid posture indicates fetal distress. A nonreactive nonstress test is consistent with acute fetal distress. Finally, inadequate amniotic fluid or no amniotic fluid indicates acute fetal distress. The biophysical profile defines inadequate amniotic fluid as the absence of amniotic fluid pockets greater than 1 cm after evaluation in two perpendicular planes.

MEASUREMENT FOR PRETERM

Sonography is a widely used method for assessing the risk of preterm delivery. This may be done by transabdominal, transperineal, or transvaginal approach. The primary goal of any sonographic approach is to assess the appearance and measurements of the cervix. The transabdominal approach is best used in a patient with a full bladder. The transperineal approach is best used with an empty bladder. The transvaginal approach is preferable and the most accurate and best used with a full bladder but carries increased risk of inducing labor, rupture of membranes, vaginal bleeding, and stimulating uterine contractions.

Sonographic measurement of the endocervical canal, by transvaginal approach, to determine cervical dilation and length is the most accurate method of determining preterm labor risks. Cervical length is measured as the distance from internal cervical os to external cervical os, including funnel length. In assessing risk, it also determines cervical competency. If first trimester sonographic findings include a vertical cervical measurement of less than 3 cm, dilation or a funneled cervical canal appearance, the likelihood of miscarriage is high. These findings in the second trimester, without concurrent ruptured membranes or uterine contractions, indicate an incompetent cervix. Sonographic evaluation of a cervix dilation >5 mm and length < 3 cm in the third trimester increases the risk of preterm labor and delivery.

Sonographer Role in Procedures

INTRAVASCULAR FETAL TRANSFUSION

Intravascular fetal transfusion is performed to treat fetal anemia, whatever its cause. To perform an intravascular fetal transfusion, a cordocentesis is performed concurrently. The ultrasound-guided cordocentesis allows for baseline and post-transfusion blood levels, especially fetal hematocrit, Rh factor determination, blood-typing and a complete blood count. This is all performed with the fetus temporarily paralyzed, as needle placement and maintenance is crucial. It is standard to use a 20 gauge, 5-inch needle to insert into the umbilical vein near the placental insertion. After a baseline blood sample is taken, an IV bolus of pancuronium bromide is given and transfusion started. Transfusion is with Rh negative, type O blood, washed and irradiated packed cells that are CMV negative, and cross-matched with maternal blood. The rate of transfusion is about 3-5 mL/min. Sonographically, transfusion appears as bright speckles. A post-transfusion hematocrit should be determined. Ultrasound monitoring should continue several minutes after the needle is withdrawn to assess blood leakage.

Fetal Diaphragmatic Hernia Repair

In utero diaphragmatic hernia repair is indicated if a large fetal herniation is diagnosed on sonography. It is also indicated due to the high fetal mortality rate of an untreated diaphragmatic herniation. Diaphragmatic herniation occurs when fetal abdominal contents press through a hole in the diaphragm into the chest cavity. This usually occurs in the posterolateral left hemidiaphragm. This leads to fetal respiratory distress and atrophied fetal lung(s). Repair of this condition is done by laparoscopy. The fetal trachea is clamped, causing the fetal lung volume to gradually increase with fluid. This increased fetal lung volume, within the thorax, pushes any herniated abdominal contents back into the abdominal cavity.

Sonohysterography

Sonohysterography involves injecting sterile saline into the uterus by using a transcervical approach to evaluate the endometrium. This method provides clinicians with even more detail than a transvaginal ultrasound. This exam may be performed to better discern abnormal findings on a pelvic ultrasound; to better evaluate the endometrium when it appears thicker than normal; or in suspected cases of endometrial polyps, submucosal fibroids, cancer, or hyperplasia; to evaluate abnormal uterine bleeding; to investigate repeated pregnancy loss; or to determine if the patient's fallopian tubes are patent. If there is a greater amount of free fluid present after the saline is injected, there is patency of at least one of the fallopian tubes. It is important to note that sonohysterography should not be performed on patients who have extreme pelvic pain, are pregnant, or who may have a pelvic infection.

A hysterosonogram should be scheduled after the patient's menstrual period, but prior to ovulation because this test should not be performed on pregnant women. Written consent should be obtained prior to the procedure with the sonographer obtaining images and measurements before the catheter is inserted. The physician performing this exam will place a speculum to access the cervix. The catheter should be flushed with sterile saline before it is inserted, and aseptic methods should be used to properly clean the cervix. Ultrasound should be used when saline is injected to demonstrate the filling of the endometrium with the appropriate images taken after the saline is injected to complete this exam. Color Doppler or 3D images may also be taken of any abnormal structures identified. The patient should be informed to contact her physician if any heavy bleeding or symptoms of infection occur afterwards.

Amniocentesis

An amniocentesis is offered in cases that have an increased risk of chromosomal defects such as mothers who are ages 35 or older or in cases of positive prenatal screenings. They may also be performed if either parent has a known genetic disorder, if there is a history of malformations in earlier pregnancies (such as neural tube defects or Down syndrome), or if an ultrasound suggested possible deformities or could not find the cause of any abnormal labs. Although this exam is typically performed to diagnose chromosomal defects, it can also determine the blood type of the fetus or evaluate the maturity of the lungs. An amniocentesis examines the amniotic fluid, which contains chemicals released by the baby as well as fetal cells to assess for any birth defects. This study should be performed after 15 weeks to avoid the risk of dry taps.

Performance Under Ultrasound Guidance

The sonographer should always make sure that written consent is obtained and questions that the patient may have about an amniocentesis are answered prior to the procedure. Associated risks should also be communicated prior to the start of the exam. Prior ultrasound exams and reports should be obtained, if any were completed. An ultrasound survey should be performed prior to the start of an amniocentesis to determine fetal position, movement, presence of cardiac activity, placental location, and largest vertical pocket of amniotic fluid (this is found with a transverse position of the probe). The operator must be sure that the transducer is perpendicular to the mother's abdomen. Sterile technique must be performed during this procedure to decrease any risk of infection. The needle must always be visualized and especially before it is inserted into the amniotic cavity. It is ideal to withdraw 20 cc of fluid that does not contain cells from the mother for proper evaluation. The amniotic fluid should be labeled and sent to the lab for analysis.

Cordocentesis

Cordocentesis is also known as percutaneous umbilical blood sampling, which is more descriptive of the technique. Cordocentesis requires an ultrasound to locate the insertion point of the umbilical cord into the placenta. With ultrasound guiding, a needle is inserted through the maternal abdomen, through the maternal uterine wall, and into the umbilical cord to collect a small sampling of cord blood. The sample is collected from the umbilical vein. Note: cordocentesis cannot be undertaken unless the fetus is immobilized by use of intramuscular fetal injection of muscle relaxant. The blood sample is then sent for laboratory analysis. Cordocentesis may be performed when other testing methods such as amniocentesis and ultrasound are inconclusive. It is performed after 17 weeks of gestation.

Chorionic Villus Sampling

Chorionic villus sampling (CVS) is a procedure that may be performed relatively early in pregnancy, between the 10th and 12th weeks. It may be performed before amniocentesis and is used to determine the sex of the baby and identify genetic problems with the fetus. Chorionic villus sampling is not generally done as a routine screening test, due to slight increase in risk of miscarriage. It is a test that is primarily considered if a fetus is suspected to be at higher risk of a specific chromosomal disorder. Chorionic villus sampling may be considered if the mother is older than age 35, she has a previous child with a chromosomal disorder, or there is a known family history of a specific genetic disorder. This test does not assess the risk of neural tube defects.

Chorionic villus sampling is an optional test done at approximately 12 weeks gestation that involves obtaining a sample of the chorion and studying it for fetal genetic abnormalities. The chorion is the fluid that surrounds the fetus and arises from the chorion villi, or the fingerlike projections that arise from the placenta. The chorion sample can be gathered by two different methods. The transcervical approach is far more common than the transabdominal approach. The decision on which approach to use is based largely on a careful pre-procedure ultrasound that identifies the exact location of the placenta and the fetal viability. Both approaches maintain ultrasound guidance while inserting a catheter into the chorionic villi of the placenta to gather the sample. Both procedures use highly aseptic conditions. The transcervical approach inserts the catheter through the vagina, cervix, and placenta to gain the sample. The transabdominal approach inserts the catheter through the maternal abdominal wall, uterus, and placenta to gather chorion.

Ultrasound Assistance for IUCD Placement

Many providers use ultrasound guidance for the placement of an IUCD. This exam will provide information regarding the size of the uterus and how it is positioned (anteverted, anteflexed, retroverted, or retroflexed). It is also important to check for congenital anomalies such as a bicornuate uterus because this is a contraindication of IUCD placement because a concurrent pregnancy, while rare, could develop in the horn opposite the device. The operator should also check for an intrauterine pregnancy; if this is seen, the device cannot be inserted. After insertion, ultrasound can be used to check for the correct location within the fundal portion of the endometrial cavity.

Diagnosing and Treating Infertility

Infertility work-up begins with a thorough history of both partners. Furthermore, it often includes physical exam, lab work, semen analysis, basal body temperature measurements, and imaging studies. Pelvic and transvaginal ultrasound may assess any anatomical abnormality or underlying disorder that may contribute to anovulation. Testicular ultrasound may be considered in some cases of male infertility evaluation. Hysterosalpingogram is widely used to assess fallopian tube patency and the uterus. Hysteroscopy allows for evaluation of endometrial cavity and any anatomical limitation of fertility. Laparoscopy may also be used in the work-up of infertility.

Sonographic Follicular Monitoring

Sonographic follicular monitoring is used in a number of assisted reproductive technology treatments. It is used to monitor women that are being treated for infertility clomiphene, insemination, and HCG. Sonographic follicular monitoring is useful for monitoring the above treatments to determine timing of inseminations, timing of cycles that cannot be monitored by the LH kit, and timing of cycles that are difficult to monitor by basal body temperatures. Furthermore, sonographic follicular monitoring is used to monitor complications of the above treatments, most notably ovarian hyperstimulation syndrome. If the ovaries are being hyperstimulated, sonography will reveal progressive ovarian enlargement and ascites in the pelvic and abdominal cavity.

Infertility Examinations and Procedures

Ultrasound is instrumental in the diagnosis and management of patients that struggle with infertility. A 3D ultrasound scan is often performed in the early stages to determine if there are any congenital malformations of the female reproductive system. It is also performed to determine if the inability to conceive stems from pathologies such as fibroids, ovarian tumors, polycystic ovaries, or even obstruction of the fallopian tubes. A sonohysterosalpingogram may be performed to discern the patency of the fallopian tubes. This procedure can also help identify abnormalities of the endometrial canal. When a woman undergoes in vitro fertilization, transvaginal ultrasound will be used to monitor the growth (and number) of follicles, to evaluate the thickness of the endometrium, and to assist during egg retrieval. Some facilities prefer ultrasound guidance during embryo transfers as well. After embryo transfer, serial ultrasound scans will be performed to determine the viability of a pregnancy and to determine the number of embryos. Anatomy scans will also be performed at approximately 18–20 weeks of gestation.

Physics and Instrumentation

Hemodynamics

Gynecology

Applications of Color Doppler When Evaluating Normal Ovaries

Sonographers should use color, power, and spectral Doppler during a pelvic ultrasound to better demonstrate any ovarian or adnexal pathology. Transvaginal ultrasound (TVUS) has provided a relatively low cost, noninvasive imaging technique. When TVUS is combined with color and/or power Doppler, improved sensitivity to the vascularity and flow within the ovary can be determined in normal and abnormal tissues. Color Doppler ultrasound can be used to demonstrate a normal flow pattern within the ovary or aid in the diagnosis of ovarian torsion. Vascularity within the ovary will change with the maturation of follicles, and arterial flow can be different in the dominant ovary when compared to the nondominant ovary. A corpus luteum will demonstrate a "ring of fire" upon color or power Doppler interrogation that reveals the physiology of this structure.

Ovarian Color and Spectral Doppler Values When Benign Ovarian Mass Is Present

The ovaries are supplied with oxygen-rich blood from the ovarian arteries. These arteries arise from the abdominal aorta just inferior to the renal arteries. However, the ovaries are considered to have a dual blood supply because the ovarian arteries join with the uterine arteries in the cornual part of the uterus. These branches can provide a collateral network of blood supply for the ovary in case either aforementioned artery becomes blocked. The ovarian veins carry blood away from the ovaries. The right ovarian vein drains blood directly into the inferior vena cava (IVC), whereas the left ovarian vein empties into the left renal vein and then continues to the IVC. Benign masses of the ovary tend to display blood flow around the peripheral margin of the mass. Spectral analysis of blood flow within a normal ovary offers data pertaining to the pulsatility index (PI) and resistivity index (RI). If the impedance is moderately high, a benign lesion is often assumed. The RI in a benign lesion is typically greater than 0.4. The PI for a benign mass tends to be greater than 1.0.

Color and Spectral Doppler Characteristics of Malignant Ovarian Masses

Malignant ovarian masses tend to have certain characteristics when compared to those that are benign. Gray-scale may show cystic components with thick walls, internal septa, and mural nodules. The borders of the mass may not be discerned well. Internal solid components may also be present, and masses that are solid are more likely to be cancerous. Color and power Doppler may demonstrate a disorganized pattern of vascularity that includes a spokelike pattern extending into the middle of the mass. A malignant lesion will typically show blood flow that has high velocity, but low impedance. If the pulsatility index is less than 1.0 and the resistivity index is less than 0.4, this suggests malignancy. Some machines enable the use of 3D power Doppler, which combines the two technologies and provides power Doppler in a 3D image. This has been useful to detect ovarian cancer earlier than the two technologies used separately, which is crucial in order for treatment to be effective.

Assessing Arteriovenous Malformations

Arteriovenous malformations (AVMs) are an uncommon phenomenon, but they can be life-threatening for the patient. They are typically congenital, but they could be the result of surgical procedures of the uterus or even cancer. An AVM may display a wide variety of appearances on a pelvic ultrasound study. They may appear as noticeable, tortuous blood vessels in the outer (perimetrium) or middle (myometrium) portions of the uterus. They may also present as a mass in the cervix or uterus. The sonographer should demonstrate that these anechoic structures are vessels by applying color Doppler to show multidirectional flow. Spectral Doppler should also be used to calculate the peak systolic velocity and resistivity index and will demonstrate increased systolic velocities and low-resistance blood flow. The operator may have a difficult time discerning arteries from veins because the venous blood flow may show patterns that are comparable to an artery. AVMs are typically treated with uterine artery embolization, but the patient's age, preservation of fertility, and the size and location of the malformation are considered.

Obstetrics

Fetal Heart Rate with M-Mode

M-mode is preferred over spectral Doppler to obtain an embryonic/fetal heart rate during an OB ultrasound exam. M-mode can provide useful information pertaining to the motion of the heart that cannot be ascertained by 2D scanning alone. The motion of heart valves and leaflets can be visualized, and variations in the thickness of the heart muscle and chambers can be detected. Cardiac arrhythmias can also be detected with M-mode echocardiography. This method will not provide an audible signal for the parents to listen to, but it is the safest choice to adhere to the "as low as reasonably achievable" principle. It is the preferred method to obtain a heart rate because the energy of the beam is spread out over the entire scan line and decreases the odds of any tissue heating. Ultrasound operators can determine the heart rate from the calculation package embedded in the machines. It is imperative that any abnormal heart rate or rhythm is properly documented.

Middle Cerebral Artery and Fetal Anemia

Evaluation of the middle cerebral artery peak systolic velocity (MCA-PSV) is a technique used with increasing frequency to manage fetal anemia. This technique has proven to be very accurate and noninvasive and carries less risk than amniocentesis and cordocentesis in fetal anemia management. When obtaining the MCA-PSV study, the fetal middle cerebral artery closest to the mother's skin should be used. The angle of blood flow to the ultrasound beam should be as close to zero degrees as possible. The middle cerebral artery should be measured as close as possible to its origin in the internal carotid artery. Record the highest peak systolic velocity and generate a curve with the MCA-PSV as a function of gestational age. These measurements are accurate up to 35 weeks gestation. The more severe the fetal anemia, the more accurate the MCA-PSV technique is. However, at a fetal hemoglobin of < 1-3 gm/dl, the MCA-PSV no longer increases.

Evaluation of Ductus Venosus

The ductus venosus (DV) is an anatomical fetal structure that enables oxygen-rich blood to pass from the placenta to the inferior vena cava. After birth, the DV will close and eventually become the ligamentum venosum. During the first trimester, it is useful to image the DV in order to assist in the diagnosis of an abnormal number of chromosomes. The assessment of the DV may provide additional information regarding anemia, possible defects in the heart, or intrauterine growth restriction in the second trimester. The DV should be examined in the superior portion of the abdomen using an oblique scan plane or midsagittal plane with the focus (and magnify) on the area where the DV unites with the umbilical vein. Doppler and spectral ultrasound should be used to determine if a normal forward flow is seen. Ultrasound operators should expect variations of blood flow within the DV during the activity of the fetus, so this is best evaluated while the fetus is inactive.

Umbilical Cord Assessment with Doppler

A normal umbilical cord transports oxygenated blood from the placenta to the fetus. The umbilical cord comprises two umbilical arteries and one vein. The arteries return deoxygenated fetal blood to the placenta to become the iliac arteries. Two umbilical arteries may be confirmed with color Doppler interrogation in the region around the fetal bladder because paired umbilical arteries will be demonstrated on both sides of the bladder. The umbilical vein conveys oxygenated blood to the fetal liver from the placenta. Doppler performed on the umbilical cord may provide pertinent information, especially when the patient experiences preeclampsia or in cases of suspected intrauterine growth restriction. The appearance of the Doppler waveform will vary depending on where the gate is placed, but measurements of impedance should be lower at the placental end of the cord and greater when measured closer to the fetus. The direction and velocity of blood flow can be measured as well as the quantity of blood flow. Doppler of the umbilical vein may provide clues related to heart failure or hypoxia.

Imaging Instruments

Maintenance of Sonographic Equipment

Guidelines for use and maintenance of sonographic equipment used to evaluate the pelvis should be known and reviewed periodically by all personal. AIUM as well as individual manufacturer guidelines should be followed. Appropriate infectious disease protocols should be recognized and applied as well. Real-time equipment with sufficient transducer frequency should be used. Transducer frequency should be adjusted to the level that allows for the least ultrasound exposure, yet yields adequate and useful results. Transducer frequency is chosen based on the unit used, the approach (transabdominal versus transvaginal), and body habitus. Thorough interpretation and documentation is necessary for quality of care and legal record-keeping purposes.

M-Mode

Motion mode (M-mode) is used mainly during cardiac imaging, and it displays the depth of echoes in regards to time represented by an *x* axis and a *y* axis. The *x* axis relates to time and is the horizontal plane. The *y* axis is a vertical axis that displays the depth of the anatomy. As the tracing moves from left to right across the screen, if the line rises up it indicates that the structure is closer to the transducer. A line that drops down is moving away from the probe, and a horizontal line means that the anatomy is not moving. M-mode offers excellent temporal resolution because data are gathered from only one ultrasound signal that is sent and received by the transducer. Even structures that are moving extremely fast can be accurately measured with M-mode. The location of the line can quickly be changed by the ultrasound operator, but care should be taken because more accurate measurements are calculated when the line is perpendicular to the structure. In addition to adult and pediatric echocardiography, M-mode is the preferred method of obtaining a fetal heart rate because less power is required, and it is also used during fetal echocardiograms.

Reject

Reject is the last process that takes place in the receiver. This function is typically offered in two forms: one that takes place automatically and one that can be controlled by the operator. The reject function enables the user to decide if low-level echoes should be displayed within the image. Sometimes, weaker signals will offer important data for a diagnosis, but clinicians do not want noise to be present on the image. Stronger signals are not affected by reject. Some ultrasound manufactures will have other names for reject, such as suppression or threshold. Reject can decrease the amount of electronic noise that may be visualized while imaging the gallbladder or urinary bladder.

Enhancement and Shadowing Artifacts

Clinicians may use ultrasound artifacts as a tool to increase diagnostic confidence. For example, if a structure is fluid filled, posterior enhancement should be visualized posterior to the cyst. Anything that is filled with fluid will appear anechoic because it has a lower attenuation rate. The surrounding tissue that is below anything that is fluid filled will appear brighter and is known as an enhancement artifact. While evaluating the ovaries, the enhancement artifact helps clinicians discern that the structure is fluid filled. Shadowing is the opposite of an enhancement artifact; this is a hypoechoic area posterior to a highly attenuating structure. This hypoechoic area prevents users from being able to see any underlying anatomy to these objects, but it provides clues of stones or calcifications. Sonographers may visualize small calcifications within the ovary, artery, or even within blood vessels.

Edge Shadowing

When a sonographer visualizes a shadow protruding from the edge of a curved structure that is parallel to the axis of the ultrasound beam, it may be referred to as an edge shadow. These artifacts are portrayed as thin, hypoechoic structures that may actually prevent a user from visualizing underlying anatomical structures. These artifacts are created from a decrease in intensity as a sound beam refracts and diverges at the same time after making contact with a curved reflector. Refraction will take place when the propagation speeds are different in the presence of oblique incidence. These artifacts are often seen when performing an ultrasound of a cyst or during a testicular scan. Other examples may include a transverse image of the gallbladder or fetal head due to the curvature of these structures.

Color Flow Imaging Applications

Red blood cells make up roughly 45% of the blood in the human circulatory system. Red blood cells supply all of the cells in the body with the necessary oxygen so they can carry out their functions. If color Doppler is applied, the reflections that are visualized are the movement of the red blood cells within the heart and blood vessels. In low-flow states, the moving blood may even be seen without turning on color Doppler. It is imperative that the user pays close attention to the color map because it will provide information pertaining to the direction the blood is moving and the velocity. If red is displayed at the top of the color map, it represents blood moving toward the transducer. If blue is on the bottom, it represents blood traveling in a direction away from the transducer.

Color Flow Imaging During Pelvic and Obstetric Exams

Color Doppler can be used during pelvic ultrasound exams to determine ovarian torsion or to provide more diagnostic information in cases in which a uterine, ovarian, or adnexal mass is identified. Color Doppler can also provide important clues as to whether a mass portrays benign or malignant color flow characteristics. Benign masses tend to demonstrate peripheral flow, whereas malignant masses tend to display feeding vessels that are more centrally located. Often, malignant tumors may show hypervascularity, because malignant tumors require a fair amount of blood flow in order to proliferate. Color Doppler is also helpful in identifying an ectopic pregnancy or corpus luteal cyst. Sonographers should remember, especially during OB exams, that color Doppler requires an increase in output power, but it can be used in conjunction with spectral analysis to sample various vessels or the umbilical cord when necessary.

Advantages and Disadvantages of Power Doppler

Power Doppler (also referred to as energy mode or color angio) is a form of color Doppler that does not display the speed of blood flow or any directional information. Rather, it only determines that a Doppler shift has taken place and shows the amplitude of the moving blood. If there are more red blood cells in one area, the signals will be brighter. Vessels represented with power Doppler will all be identical colors on the display. Advantages of power Doppler include the fact that aliasing does not occur because the speed and direction of blood flow is not applicable. Power Doppler picks up blood flow in smaller vessels and slow blood flow because of its increase in sensitivity. There is an increase in sensitivity because power Doppler is not altered by the Doppler angle. A disadvantage of power Doppler is that, due to the increased sensitivity, flash artifact may be visualized when the patient moves or breathes. Power Doppler does not evaluate the direction or velocity of blood flow. When compared to color Doppler, the temporal resolution is greatly reduced.

Pulsed-Wave Doppler

Pulsed-wave Doppler is used to calculate the velocity of red blood cells that are moving within various blood vessels. From these calculations, the peak systole, end diastole, pulsatility index, and resistive index can be calculated; they provide useful information to clinicians pertaining to any pathology. The ultrasound user can choose the exact location where the measurements should be taken by placing the gate within the lumen of the vessel. The gate size can be adjusted if necessary, to get a more precise measurement. Aliasing may be a concern when using pulsed-wave Doppler, so the user may need to adjust the scale or depth of the anatomical structure being imaged, switch to a transducer with a lower frequency, or switch to continuous-wave Doppler. If the velocities are too high to be accurately measured, then the user should switch to continuous-wave Doppler to obtain the maximum velocity.

Spectral Analysis

Spectral analysis is the technique used during pulsed Doppler to provide information pertaining to the various velocities obtained in the blood vessel or organ. Blood doesn't travel in the same direction or speed even when contained in the same sample volume. The spectral analysis window will allow clinicians to examine how the frequency shifts are dispersed within the Doppler signal. Two types of spectral analysis that are used are the fast Fourier transform (FFT) and autocorrelation. FFT is the method used to operate the spectral analysis during pulsed-wave and continuous-wave Doppler. This method can determine if the flow pattern is turbulent or if it is normal (laminar) flow. Autocorrelation is only used during color Doppler, but it is faster than the FFT method. The gate can be moved until it is where the user wants to perform a spectral analysis. The size of the gate can be changed so that it is only within the vessel that is being examined. For example, if one is sampling the carotid artery, but the spectral display is also showing venous flow, the technician will reduce the size of the gate and reposition it so only the artery is being interrogated.

Harmonics

Harmonic imaging is offered by modern ultrasound systems to improve the diagnostic capabilities, especially during exams that are technically difficult. When the harmonics application is in use, the fundamental (transmitted) frequency offers improved diagnostic quality because the beam is altered less. The ultrasound harmonics are produced within the anatomical tissue of the patient. Tissue and contrast are two common types of harmonics used. Harmonics are useful during exams to help eliminate reflectors seen inside of cysts and side-lobe artifacts. Harmonic tissue applications used during OB ultrasounds are especially useful in the second trimester to provide improved visualization of organs and other anatomy, especially when the patient is obese. The use of tissue harmonics has especially increased the resolution of the heart or when the user would like to rid the image of any associated noise.

3D Imaging

The majority of measurements during an OB ultrasound are still obtained during a 2D B-mode exam, but 3D and 4D technologies offer improved diagnostic confidence because more detail is provided than ever before. Contrast resolution is greatly improved when using 2D array transducers because they offer a thin slice thickness of the ultrasound beam. When the beam is not any wider than the anatomy being examined, it improves the contrast resolution. The use of 3D and 4D imaging during an OB exam includes imaging the fetal heart, spine, diaphragmatic hernias, extremities, lungs, and fetal face as just some of the anatomical structures that are better visualized. The 3D ultrasound offers yet another dimension to the traditional 2D exam, and 4D ultrasound is real-time 3D. Along with the diagnostic importance of 3D and 4D studies, these applications can offer parents and family a chance to bond with their baby because they can offer a more lifelike picture.

The ALARA Principle

Sonographers should implement the ALARA principle during all sonographic exams. This is especially important during an obstetric (OB) ultrasound to prevent tissue heating and the possibility of bioeffects. ALARA is an acronym that stands for as low as reasonably achievable. Ultrasound should only be used when ordered by a physician to provide pertinent clinical data. Another way that sonographers can adhere to the ALARA principle is to limit the amount of time that a patient is exposed to the sound waves and never leave the transducer in the same place on the patient for too long. The output used to create diagnostic images should be kept as low as possible. For example, if an entire image is too bright, the most effective way to decrease the patient's exposure is to decrease the output (acoustic) power. When there is a reduction in the power setting, there is a decrease in the voltage applied to the transducer, which, in turn, decreases the amount of exposure to the patient. Pulsed Doppler should only be used when necessary during OB scans because it also increases the risk of patient exposure.

Thermal Index

The thermal index (TI) refers to the ratio of power imparted on tissue that causes the temperature to rise by 1 °C. The TI is displayed as a number on the screen for sonographers as an indicator of a possible escalation of tissue temperature when sound waves are absorbed. A value of 1 equates an increase of 1 °C; ideally, the value should be less than 1. Sonographers should be cognizant of the TI during an OB exam because this is directly related to the acoustic output of the machine. There are three types of TIs that serve as the best in vivo indicators of a rise in temperature: the soft tissue TI (TIS), bone TI (TIB), and cranial bone TI (TIC). The TIB value is assumed when a patient is 10 weeks pregnant. The TIS value should be used when performing early OB scans before 10 weeks.

Mechanical Index

The mechanical index (MI) reading on an ultrasound machine determines the probability of bioeffects when gas bubbles in the tissue interact with the ultrasound beam. This is a phenomenon known as cavitation, and there are two types: stable and transient (inertial). The latter occurs with higher MI readouts and increases the risk of bursting microbubbles that can lead to an increase of temperature and pressure. A high MI offers a better chance that bioeffects will occur. If a sonographer notices that the MI is too high, it is helpful to decrease the output power on the machine. The frequency of the transducer could also be increased because frequency and MI have an inverse relationship.

ARDMS Practice Test

1. Which of the following is an indication for sonohysterography?

a. Active bleeding
b. Pelvic inflammatory disease
c. Focal endometrial thickening
d. Pregnancy

2. Uterine arteries display:

a. Lower resistance flow in postmenopausal women than in reproductive-age women.
b. Higher resistance flow in postmenopausal women than in reproductive-age women.
c. Higher resistance flow in reproductive-age women and postmenopausal women.
d. Lower resistance flow in reproductive-age women and postmenopausal women.

3. An intrauterine device may display which type of artifact with transvaginal evaluation?

a. Acoustic shadowing
b. Mirror image
c. Enhancement
d. Side lobe

4. Which transducer would best visualize a 6-week intrauterine pregnancy?

a. Sector 5.0 MHz
b. Endovaginal 12.0 MHz
c. Curvilinear 3.5 MHz
d. Linear array 17.0 MHz

5. Cervical length is considered within normal limits during pregnancy when it measures:

a. 2.5cm or greater.
b. 3.0 cm or greater.
c. 1.6 to 2.5cm.
d. 1.6cm or less.

6. Which of the following describes the formula to calculate ovarian volume?

a. 0.751 x length x width x height
b. 0.751 + length + width + height
c. 0.523 x length x width x height
d. 0.523 + length + width + height

7. All of the following statements are true regarding femur length except:

a. The femur is measured to assess fetal growth from 14 to 40 weeks.
b. The clinician should include the long axis of the ossified diaphysis in measurement.
c. If measured two standard deviations below the mean, short limb dysplasia may be considered.
d. The clinician should include the cartilaginous epiphysis in the measurement.

8. Crown-to-rump length is used to calculate gestational age by which of the following formulas?

a. CRL (cm) + 40 = GA (days)
b. CRL (cm) + 42 = GA (days)
c. CRL (mm) + 40 = GA (days)
d. CRL (mm) + 42 = GA (days)

9. A rapid decline in HCG levels may indicate which of the following scenarios?

a. Anembryonic pregnancy
b. Missed abortion
c. Incomplete abortion
d. Complete abortion

10. Elevation of CA125 may indicate which type of ovarian pathology?

a. Metastatic ovarian tumors
b. Epithelial cell tumors
c. Germ cell tumors
d. Stromal cell tumors

11. Evaluation of the peak systolic velocity of the middle cerebral artery may diagnose:

a. Fetal hydrops.
b. Oligohydramnios.
c. Fetal anemia.
d. Erythroblastosis fetalis.

12. Which of the following may enhance the evaluation of an endometrial polyp during a sonohysterogram?

a. Harmonic imaging
b. 2-D imaging
c. 3-D imaging
d. Doppler imaging

13. A 67-year-old female presents for an ultrasound of the pelvis. The patient has a history of left-sided breast cancer and has had a bilateral mastectomy. The patent has no pelvic complaints. Sonographically a thickened, heterogeneous endometrium is visualized. The most likely explanation for this appearance may include which of the following?

a. History of endometrial ablation
b. Patient is still having menstrual cycles
c. Patient has endometriosis
d. Patient is taking tamoxifen

14. Sonographic evaluation of the endometrium during the secretory phase may display which of the following?

a. Thin, slightly irregular endometrium
b. Thickened, isoechoic endometrium
c. Maximum AP diameter of 8mm
d. Thickened, hyperechoic endometrium

15. The narrowest portion of the fallopian tube is the:

a. Intramural portion.
b. Isthmus portion.
c. Ampulla portion.
d. Fimbria portion.

16. A benign tumor of the uterine musculature is best described as which of the following?

a. Nabothian cyst
b. Leiomyoma
c. Gartner's cyst
d. Adenomyosis

17. A fibroid arising from a stalk can be described as:

a. Pedunculated.
b. Exophytic.
c. Submucosal.
d. Subserous.

18. A biophysical profile examines all of the following sonographically except:

a. The fetal non-stress test.
b. Gross body movements.
c. Fetal breathing.
d. Fetal tone.

19. Blood is shunted from the right to left atrium in the fetal heart through which cardiac structure?

a. Semi-lunar valve
b. Ductus arteriosus
c. Mitral valve
d. Foramen ovale

20. All of the following structures are measured in the assessment of fetal weight except:

a. Biparietal diameter.
b. Femur length.
c. Humerus length.
d. Head circumference.

21. A 15-year-old female presents to the ultrasound department for a pelvic evaluation for secondary amenorrhea. The patient is not sexually active. What is the proper patient prep for her pelvic ultrasound?

a. The patient should void several minutes prior to her exam
b. The patient should drink 24 to 32 oz of water one hour prior to the exam and should not void
c. The patient should drink 24 to 32 oz of water upon arriving to her appointment and should not void
d. There is no prep necessary for her pelvic ultrasound

22. A 38-year-old patient presents to the ultrasound department for growth, fluid, and fetal position assessment. By her LMP, the fetal gestational age is determined to be 33 weeks and 2 days. The patient has a history of smoking and diabetes. In the sonographic evaluation to rule out intrauterine growth restriction, what is expected?

a. Macrocephaly
b. Oligohydramnios
c. Stage 2 placenta
d. Large for gestational age

23. A patient presents to the ultrasound department with menorrhagia. This means the patient is experiencing which of the following?

a. An excessive amount of bleeding during menstruation
b. An abnormally small amount of bleeding during menstruation
c. Painful bleeding during menstruation
d. The absence of bleeding during menstruation

24. During a second trimester fetal sonogram the placenta is evaluated. The sonographer demonstrates an increase in the myometrial echogenicity and thickness near the site of the placenta. Which of the following may be considered?

a. Placenta previa
b. Placenta increta
c. Placenta percreta
d. Placenta accreta

25. The sonographic evaluation for fetal position demonstrates a fetus in the breech position with the hips extended and feet presenting. This is known as which of the following?

a. Shoulder breech
b. Frank breech
c. Footling breech
d. Complete breech

26. The fundus, body, and cervix of the uterus are tilted posteriorly in relation to the vagina. What is the described uterine position?

a. Retroflexed
b. Retroverted
c. Dextroverted
d. Levorotated

27. Which of the following is true regarding the biparietal diameter?

a. It is measured at the level of the thalami and cavum septum
b. It is measured at the level of the cerebellum and posterior fossa
c. It is measured from one outer parietal bone to the other outer parietal bone
d. It is measured at the level of the lateral ventricles and choroid plexus

28. A 17-year-old presents for her 20-week fetal anomaly screening. Sonographically, loops of bowel are seen extending into the amniotic cavity. The bowel appears to be protruding from the abdominal wall to the right of the cord insertion. There appears to be no membrane enclosing the loops of bowel. The most likely diagnosis would be which of the following?

a. Omphalocele
b. Encephalocele
c. Normal bowel herniation
d. Gastroschisis

29. A 34-year-old female presents with a history of infertility. Sonographically, a unicornuate uterus is demonstrated. What other organ should be evaluated upon discovery of this anomaly?

a. Liver
b. Spleen
c. Pancreas
d. Kidneys

30. Which of the following hormones stimulates maturation and ovulation of the Graafian follicle?

a. Follicle-stimulating hormone
b. Luteinizing hormone
c. Estrogen
d. Progesterone

31. What portion of the lateral ventricle is measured during a fetal anomaly screening?

a. Atrium
b. Anterior horn
c. Body
d. Posterior horn

32. A greater than expected hCG level may indicate all of the following except:

a. Embryonic demise.
b. Incorrect dates.
c. Gestational trophoblastic disease.
d. Multiple gestations.

33. A patient complains of pelvic pain and spotting. Her hCG levels were 1200mIU/mL. Sonographically, there is free fluid in the cul-de-sac, an endometrial decidual reaction, and a complex area demonstrated in the adnexa. What is the most likely diagnosis?

a. Normal intrauterine pregnancy
b. Gestational trophoblastic disease
c. Ectopic pregnancy
d. Corpus luteum cyst

34. A 17-year-old female presents for a viability sonogram. By her LMP, she should be 13 weeks and 4 days. The patient complains of hyperemesis, pelvic fullness, and bloating. The HCG levels are grossly elevated. Sonographically, a soft tissue-like mass fills the endometrial cavity. The mass appears heterogeneous, and is described as having a snowstorm appearance. What is the most likely diagnosis?

a. Choriocarcinoma
b. Invasive mole
c. Partial mole
d. Complete hydatidiform mole

35. Which of the following ligaments attaches the cornua of the uterus to the anterior pelvic wall?

a. Ovarian
b. Broad
c. Round
d. Cardinal

36. Which of the following best describes intrauterine insemination?

a. Embryos are developed outside of the body and are delivered into the uterus through a catheter
b. Embryos are developed outside of the body and are placed into the fallopian tube
c. Both parents' gametes are placed within the fallopian tube
d. The male gamete is inserted into the fundus of the uterus with a catheter

37. A didelphys and bicornuate uterus are congenital anomalies of the uterus that occur due to the:

a. Failure of formation.
b. Failure of fusion.
c. Failure of dissolution.
d. Failure of disappearance.

38. The normal evaluation of the genitourinary system includes evaluation of all of the following structures except the:

a. Kidneys.
b. Stomach.
c. Bladder.
d. Adrenal glands.

39. A patient is 18 weeks and 5 days pregnant. She presents to the ultrasound department for a fetal anomaly screening. The renal pelvis is seen and measured. What are the normal limits of the AP measurement of the renal pelvis at this age of pregnancy?

a. Less than 2mm
b. Less than or equal to 5 mm
c. 5 to 10mm
d. Greater than or equal to 10 mm

40. A fetus demonstrates frontal bossing of the cranium. The cerebellum is dislocated and there is obliteration of the cistern magna. What is a likely diagnosis?

a. Spina bifida
b. Anencephaly
c. Iniencephaly
d. Encephalocele

41. Sonographic evaluation of the fetal cranium demonstrates a large cystic space. The face is also evaluated and demonstrates proboscis and cyclopia. What is the most likely diagnosis?

a. Hydranencephaly
b. Porencephaly
c. Hydrocephaly
d. Holoprosencephaly

42. Which type of osteogenesis imperfecta is lethal?

a. Type 1
b. Type 2
c. Type 3
d. Type 4

43. All of the following are true regarding twin-to-twin transfusion syndrome except:

a. It occurs with monozygotic/monochorionic twins.
b. There is an artery-to-vein anastomosis that shunts blood away from the donor twin to the recipient twin.
c. The donor twin measures large for dates.
d. The recipient twin may demonstrate polyhydramnios.

44. All of the following may be typically visualized sonographically in a patient with gestational diabetes except:

a. IUGR.
b. Macrosomia.
c. A single umbilical artery.
d. A thickened placenta.

45. Hematometra displays as which of the following?

a. Pus in the uterus
b. Water in the uterus
c. Blood in the vagina
d. Blood in the uterus

46. The umbilical cord is made up of:

a. One artery and two veins.
b. One artery and one vein.
c. Two arteries and one vein.
d. Two arteries and two veins.

47. Evaluation of the right ovary demonstrates sonographic evidence of a highly echogenic mass that displays shadowing and obscures the posterior wall of the mass. What is the most likely diagnosis?

a. Dermoid tumor
b. Dysgerminoma
c. Yolk sac tumor
d. Fibroma

48. A patient presents for a pelvic ultrasound. She complains of fever, lower abdominal pain, and vaginal discharge. Her labs indicate leukocytosis. What is a likely diagnosis?

a. Endometriosis
b. Pelvic congestion syndrome
c. Urinary tract infection
d. Pelvic inflammatory disease

49. All of the following are true regarding trisomy 21 except:

a. It is also known as Down syndrome.
b. It is also known as Edward's syndrome.
c. It may be present if the nuchal fold measures greater than 6mm between 15 to 21 weeks' gestation.
d. Intellectual disability and abnormal physical characteristics may be present.

50. Fetal evaluation demonstrates macroglossia, gigantism, cardiac malformations, and placental enlargement. What is a likely diagnosis?

a. Pentalogy of Cantrell
b. Meckel-Gruber syndrome
c. Beckwith-Wiedemann syndrome
d. VATER association

Answer Key and Explanations

1. C: Focal endometrial thickening

Sonohysterography is saline-infused sonography. Saline is infused through a placed catheter within the endometrial cavity to outline the cavity. This exam is typically performed to rule out endometrial abnormalities such as an endometrial polyp that may be seen as focal endometrial thickening on a typical sonogram. Pregnancy, PID, and active bleeding are all contraindications of this exam. Though abnormal bleeding may be an indication for the exam, active bleeding may prevent the radiologist from performing the exam. The risk of infection increases and false positive results may occur if performed on a patient with active bleeding.

2. B: Higher resistance flow in postmenopausal women than in reproductive-age women

The uterine arteries display higher resistance flow in postmenopausal women than in reproductive-age women. Postmenopausal women are no longer having menstrual cycles. Therefore, the resistance of the uterine arteries no longer has to decrease during the luteal phase of the menstrual cycle. The arteries remain at a higher resistance because they no longer need to function for the purposes of reproduction. A woman of reproductive age will display lower resistance of the uterine arteries since her uterus is still functioning for the purpose of preparing each month for a possible pregnancy.

3. A: Acoustic shadowing

An intrauterine device may display acoustic shadowing when evaluated with transvaginal sonography. Shadowing is the reduction in echo amplitude from reflectors that lie posterior to a strongly reflecting structure such as an IUD. The echoes posterior to the strongly reflecting IUD will appear darker, such as a shadow.

4. B: Endovaginal 12.0 MHz

An endovaginal 12.0 MHz transducer will best visualize a 6-week intrauterine pregnancy. Early pregnancies are best visualized endovaginally. A fetal pole and heart rate may be visualized 1 to 2 weeks earlier than when using a curvilinear transducer. It may also provide more precise dating calculations due to the better resolution and magnified view than a curvilinear or sector probe can provide. A linear array 17.0 MHz probe is more likely to be used for the evaluation of superficial structures within the breast tissue.

5. A: 2.5cm or greater

The cervical length is considered within normal limits during pregnancy when it measures 2.5cm or greater. An incompetent cervix is considered when it measures less than 2.5cm. A cervix that measures 1.6 to 2.5cm in length is considered incompetent and the patient may be required to decrease physical activity or be put on bed rest. When the cervical length is less than 1.6cm, a cerclage may be surgically applied to the cervix. If a cervix is incompetent, there is a risk for premature labor.

6. C: 0.523 x length x width x height

The formula to calculate ovarian volume is 0.523 x length x width x height. A patient who is premenopausal may have an ovarian volume that ranges with ovulatory stage, between $5.1cm^3$-$3.2cm^3$. A postmenopausal patient may also have a range of ovarian volume depending on her number of years past menopause, $1.3cm^3$. Ovarian volume is the preferred method for determining ovarian size.

7. D: the clinician should include the cartilaginous epiphysis in the measurement.

The femur length should be measured in the long axis of the ossified portion of the diaphysis and should not include the cartilaginous epiphysis in the measurement. Femur length is used to help determine fetal weight and growth. If the femur length is measured two standard deviations below the mean, short limb dysplasia may be considered and other long bones of the body should be evaluated.

8. D: CRL (mm) + 42 = GA (days)

The correct formula for calculating gestational age is CRL (mm) + 42 = GA (days). Crown-to-rump length (CRL) is the most accurate measurement for dating throughout pregnancy. It is measured from the top of the fetal head to bottom of the rump, excluding any limbs. CRL is measured between 6- and 11-weeks' gestation.

9. D: Complete abortion

A rapid decline in HCG levels may indicate a complete abortion. A complete abortion is complete evacuation of all products of the pregnancy. The HCG levels will decline rapidly and the pregnancy symptoms will no longer be present. During an anembryonic pregnancy, the hCG levels are variable. They may rise at a normal rate but then plateau or decrease. A missed abortion may demonstrate less than expected HCG levels. An incomplete abortion may display a slow decrease or plateau of the HCG levels.

10. B: Epithelial cell tumor

Elevation of the tumor marker CA125 may indicate an epithelial cell tumor. It is elevated in about 80% of women with epithelial ovarian cancer. Unfortunately, it may not be detected in stage 1 of this cancer. The tumor marker CA125 may also be elevated in the bloodstream of a woman who has fibroids or endometriosis.

11. C: Fetal anemia

The evaluation of the peak systolic velocity of the middle cerebral artery may diagnose fetal anemia. With the evaluation of the MCA, there has been a decreased need for invasive procedures, which has reduced the rate of fetal death in utero.

12. C: 3-D imaging

3-D imaging may enhance the evaluation of an endometrial polyp during a sonohysterogram. 3-D imaging obtains a volume render that can be saved and later reconstructed. The reconstructed coronal view may display the size, number, shape, and location of the polyp.

13. D: Patient is taking tamoxifen

A patient with a history of breast cancer and who displays a thickened, heterogeneous endometrium on the sonogram may be taking tamoxifen. Tamoxifen is an estrogen-blocking medication of the breast but an estrogen stimulator of the pelvis. It is prescribed to many patients who have had breast cancer that tested positive for estrogen stimulation. The downside is that the medication may cause proliferation of the endometrium, which is why it is important to take a good patient history prior to the ultrasound.

14. D: Thickened, hyperechoic endometrium

Sonographic evaluation of the endometrium during the secretory phase may display a thickened, hyperechoic endometrium. The endometrium may display posterior enhancement and may measure up to 18mm in AP diameter. The secretory phase occurs during days 15 to 28. A thin, slightly irregular endometrium may be seen during the menstrual phase. A thickened, isoechoic endometrium with a max AP of 8mm may be seen during the proliferative phase.

15. A: Intramural portion

The narrowest portion of the fallopian tube is the intramural portion. It is located within the cornu of the uterus. The isthmus is located between the intramural and the ampulla portion. The ampulla is the longest portion of tube. It extends into the fimbria, which catches the released eggs.

16. B: Leiomyoma

A leiomyoma is a benign tumor of the uterine musculature. It is more commonly seen in African American women. A nabothian cyst is a cyst seen within the cervix. A Gartner's duct cyst is seen within the vagina. Adenomyosis is a benign diffuse disease where the endometrial stroma invades the myometrium.

17. A: Pedunculated

A fibroid arising from a stalk can be described as pedunculated. An exophytic fibroid grows out of the uterus. Submucosal fibroids press against the endometrium. Subserous fibroids are located close to the outer peritoneal surface of the uterus.

18. A: the fetal non-stress test

Sonographically, a biophysical profile evaluates fetal breathing for at least 30 seconds, at least three gross body movements, and at least one episode of fetal tone within 30 minutes scanning time. A fetal non-stress test score may be added into the total score of the BPP, but it is not a sonographic evaluation. AFI may also be included in the score.

19. D: Foramen ovale

Blood is shunted from the right to left atrium in the fetal heart through the foramen ovale. After birth, the foramen ovale should close.

20. C: Humerus length

Biparietal diameter, femur length, head circumference, and abdominal circumference are all measured in the assessment of fetal weight. Humerus length may be measured to assess fetal age.

21. B: the patient should drink 24 to 32 oz of water one hour prior to the exam and should not void

Given the patient's age and sexual history, the evaluation of her pelvis will be performed trans-abdominally. The patient prep for a trans-abdominal ultrasound involves the patient drinking 24 to 32 oz of water one hour prior to exam and she should not void. A full bladder produces a window for the evaluation of the uterus and the endometrium.

22. B: Oligohydramnios

Intrauterine growth restriction may present sonographically with oligohydramnios, advanced maturity of the placenta, microcephaly, and small for gestational age. Asymmetrical IUGR is the most common type. The fetal head is not in proportion with the fetal body because the blood supply is being sent to the brain, restricting growth of the rest of the body. The abdominal circumference measures more than 2 weeks behind the head circumference.

23. A: an excessive amount of bleeding during menstruation

Menorrhagia is an excessive amount of bleeding during menstruation. Hypomenorrhea is an abnormally small amount of bleeding during menstruation. Dysmenorrhea is painful bleeding during menstruation. Amenorrhea is the absence of bleeding during menstruation.

24. C: Placenta percreta

Placenta increta, percreta, and accreta are defined as the abnormal adherence of the placenta to the uterine wall. Placenta percreta appears sonographically as an increase in the myometrial echogenicity and thickness. It occurs when the placental tissue invades through the myometrium. Placenta increta is the deep invasion of the placental tissue within the myometrium. Placenta accreta is the attachment of the placenta villi to the myometrium. Placenta previa is defined by the location of the placenta in relation to the cervical internal os.

25. C: Footling breech

Breech position is when the fetal head is visualized in the fundus of the uterus. Footling breech occurs when the fetal hips are extended and the feet are presenting. Frank breech occurs when the fetal hips are flexed and the knees are extended. Complete breech occurs when the fetal hips and the knees are flexed. Shoulder presentation occurs when the shoulders are presenting.

26. B: Retroverted

Retroverted uterine position is described when the fundus, body, and cervix of the uterus are tilted posteriorly. Retroflexed uterine position is displayed as the fundus and body of the uterus tilted posterior in relation to the cervix. Dextroverted uterine position is displayed as deviation of the long axis of the uterus and cervix to the right of midline.

Levorotated is described as the deviation of the uterus and cervix in the long axis to the left of midline.

27. A: It is measured at the level of the thalami and cavum septum

The biparietal diameter is measured at the level of the thalami and cavum septum. The calipers for a proper measurement are from the most anterior outer parietal bone to the inner parietal bone.

28. D: Gastroschisis

Gastroschisis is displayed sonographically as bowel herniation into the amniotic cavity. There is no membrane that covers the bowel and it's usually seen protruding from the right of the cord insertion. Normal bowel herniation may be seen from 8 to 12 weeks' gestation; therefore, the patient is too far along for that to be considered in this situation. An omphalocele is similar to gastroschisis but the bowel is contained within a membrane. An encephalocele is seen in the brain when the brain tissue protrudes from the posterior fossa.

29. D: Kidneys

Upon discovery of a unicornuate uterus, the sonographer should also evaluate the kidneys. Both the uterus and the kidneys develop from the müllerian duct. There is a possibility of a renal anomaly such as renal agenesis.

30. B: Luteinizing hormone

Luteinizing hormone (LH) stimulates maturation and ovulation of the Graafian follicle. A decreased level of estradiol stimulates the hypothalamus to release gonadotropin-releasing hormone (GnRH). GnRH stimulates the pituitary gland to release follicle-stimulating hormone (FSH) and LH. FSH stimulates the growth and development of ovarian follicles. The increasing size of the follicles causes an increase in estrogen levels. With the development of the corpus luteum by LH stimulation of the ovary, progesterone increases and peaks right after ovulation. When a pregnancy occurs, HCG signals the corpus luteum to prevent menstruation. If no pregnancy has occurred, progesterone levels drop and the endometrial lining is shed.

31. A: Atrium

The atrium is the portion of the lateral ventricle that is measured during a fetal anomaly screening.

32. A: Embryonic demise

Greater than expected HCG levels may indicate incorrect dates, gestational trophoblastic disease, and multiple gestations. Embryonic demise would demonstrate less than expected HCG levels.

33. C: Ectopic pregnancy

The most likely diagnosis is an ectopic pregnancy. When the HCG levels are at least 800-1000 mIU/mL, more than just an endometrial decidual reaction should be visualized. A gestational sac should be visualized when the HCG levels are 1200 mIU/mL. Free fluid in the cul-de-sac may be seen with an ectopic pregnancy. Sometimes a complex mass similar to the appearance of a corpus luteum cyst can be seen in the adnexa, demonstrating an ectopic pregnancy.

34. D: Complete hydatidiform mole

A complete hydatidiform mole is the most common type of gestational trophoblastic disease. A complete mole will demonstrate a heterogeneous mass filling the endometrium sonographically. Partial mole is associated with triploid. It transforms the placenta and causes severe IUGR. It is lethal to the pregnancy. Invasive mole will invade the myometrium. Choriocarcinoma is a highly metastatic tumor.

35. C: Round

The round ligament attaches the cornua of the uterus to the anterior pelvic wall. It is located anterior and inferior to the broad ligaments and fallopian tubes. The ovarian ligament attaches the ovary to the uterine cornu. The broad ligament extends from the lateral aspect of the uterus to the lateral pelvic walls. The cardinal ligaments are the primary support of the uterus. They course superiorly and laterally from the uterus and arise inferiorly from the vagina.

36. D: the male gamete is inserted into the fundus of the uterus with a catheter

IUI is best described as the male gamete being inserted into the fundus of the uterus with a catheter.

37. B: Failure of fusion

A didelphys and bicornuate uterus are congenital anomalies of the uterus that occur due to the failure of fusion.

38. B: Stomach

The stomach is part of the gastrointestinal system. The kidneys, bladder, and adrenal glands are part of the genitourinary system. All structures should be evaluated sonographically.

39. B: Less than or equal to 5mm

The normal renal pelvis measurement for a fetus between 13- and 20-weeks' gestational age is 5 mm.

40. A: Spina bifida

Spina bifida occurs due to the lack of closure of the spinal vertebral column. Intracranial sonographic evaluation may demonstrate the lemon sign and the banana sign. Iniencephaly sonographically demonstrates as a hyperextended fetal head. Encephalocele appears sonographically where the brain tissue is herniated outside of the skull. Anencephaly sonographically demonstrates the absence of portions of the fetal cranium and intracranial structures.

41. D: Holoprosencephaly

Holoprosencephaly may demonstrate sonographically as a large midline cystic space. The face may display a proboscis and cyclopia. There are three types of holoprosencephaly which are alobar, semilobar, and lobar.

42. B: Type 2

Osteogenesis imperfecta may result in fractured limbs, limb bowing, and bruising. Types 1 and 4 have the best prognosis. Type 2 is lethal.

43. C: the donor twin measures large for dates

When twin-to-twin transfusion syndrome is present, the donor twin will present as small for dates. Blood is shunted away from the donor twin to the recipient twin through an artery-to-vein anastomosis. The recipient twin may demonstrate polyhydramnios, but the donor twin may display severe oligohydramnios. This syndrome occurs with monozygotic/monochorionic twins.

44. A: IUGR

IUGR may be seen sonographically in patients with gestational hypertension. Patients with gestational diabetes may demonstrate fetal macrosomia, a single umbilical artery, and a thickened placenta.

45. D: Blood in the uterus

Hematometra is blood in the uterus. Pyometra is pus in the uterus. Hydrometra is water in the uterus. Hematocolpos is blood in the vagina.

46. C: Two arteries and one vein

The umbilical cord is made up of two arteries and one vein. The arteries carry deoxygenated blood away from the fetus and the vein carries oxygenated blood to the fetus.

47. A: Dermoid tumor

Dermoids are the most common benign germ cell tumor. They may display the tip of the iceberg sign sonographically. They may cause ovarian torsion.

48. D: Pelvic inflammatory disease

The patient with PID may complain of symptoms of infection. With the labs being positive for increased white blood cells, the most likely diagnosis is PID.

49. B: It is also known as Edward's syndrome

Edward's syndrome is known as trisomy 18. Down syndrome is trisomy 21. Patau's syndrome is trisomy 13.

50. C: Beckwith-Wiedemann syndrome

Beckwith-Wiedemann syndrome is associated with macroglossia, gigantism, omphalocele, cardiac malformations, and placental enlargement. It may be known as an overgrowth syndrome. Children with this syndrome have a chance of developing a cancerous tumor known as Wilms' tumor. They are also at risk for the development of liver cancer known as hepatoblastoma. Pentalogy of Cantrell is associated with an omphalocele and ectopic cordis. Meckel-Gruber syndrome is associated with encephalocele, polycystic kidneys, cleft lip, and polydactyly. VATER association or VACTERL stands for vertebral anomalies, anal atresia, cardiac anomalies, tracheoesophageal atresia, renal anomalies, and limb anomalies.

How to Overcome Test Anxiety

Just the thought of taking a test is enough to make most people a little nervous. A test is an important event that can have a long-term impact on your future, so it's important to take it seriously and it's natural to feel anxious about performing well. But just because anxiety is normal, that doesn't mean that it's helpful in test taking, or that you should simply accept it as part of your life. Anxiety can have a variety of effects. These effects can be mild, like making you feel slightly nervous, or severe, like blocking your ability to focus or remember even a simple detail.

If you experience test anxiety—whether severe or mild—it's important to know how to beat it. To discover this, first you need to understand what causes test anxiety.

Causes of Test Anxiety

While we often think of anxiety as an uncontrollable emotional state, it can actually be caused by simple, practical things. One of the most common causes of test anxiety is that a person does not feel adequately prepared for their test. This feeling can be the result of many different issues such as poor study habits or lack of organization, but the most common culprit is time management. Starting to study too late, failing to organize your study time to cover all of the material, or being distracted while you study will mean that you're not well prepared for the test. This may lead to cramming the night before, which will cause you to be physically and mentally exhausted for the test. Poor time management also contributes to feelings of stress, fear, and hopelessness as you realize you are not well prepared but don't know what to do about it.

Other times, test anxiety is not related to your preparation for the test but comes from unresolved fear. This may be a past failure on a test, or poor performance on tests in general. It may come from comparing yourself to others who seem to be performing better or from the stress of living up to expectations. Anxiety may be driven by fears of the future—how failure on this test would affect your educational and career goals. These fears are often completely irrational, but they can still negatively impact your test performance.

Elements of Test Anxiety

As mentioned earlier, test anxiety is considered to be an emotional state, but it has physical and mental components as well. Sometimes you may not even realize that you are suffering from test anxiety until you notice the physical symptoms. These can include trembling hands, rapid heartbeat, sweating, nausea, and tense muscles. Extreme anxiety may lead to fainting or vomiting. Obviously, any of these symptoms can have a negative impact on testing. It is important to recognize them as soon as they begin to occur so that you can address the problem before it damages your performance.

The mental components of test anxiety include trouble focusing and inability to remember learned information. During a test, your mind is on high alert, which can help you recall information and stay focused for an extended period of time. However, anxiety interferes with your mind's natural processes, causing you to blank out, even on the questions you know well. The strain of testing during anxiety makes it difficult to stay focused, especially on a test that may take several hours. Extreme anxiety can take a huge mental toll, making it difficult not only to recall test information but even to understand the test questions or pull your thoughts together.

Effects of Test Anxiety

Test anxiety is like a disease—if left untreated, it will get progressively worse. Anxiety leads to poor performance, and this reinforces the feelings of fear and failure, which in turn lead to poor performances on subsequent tests. It can grow from a mild nervousness to a crippling condition. If allowed to progress, test anxiety can have a big impact on your schooling, and consequently on your future.

Test anxiety can spread to other parts of your life. Anxiety on tests can become anxiety in any stressful situation, and blanking on a test can turn into panicking in a job situation. But fortunately, you don't have to let anxiety rule your testing and determine your grades. There are a number of relatively simple steps you can take to move past anxiety and function normally on a test and in the rest of life.

Physical Steps for Beating Test Anxiety

While test anxiety is a serious problem, the good news is that it can be overcome. It doesn't have to control your ability to think and remember information. While it may take time, you can begin taking steps today to beat anxiety.

Just as your first hint that you may be struggling with anxiety comes from the physical symptoms, the first step to treating it is also physical. Rest is crucial for having a clear, strong mind. If you are tired, it is much easier to give in to anxiety. But if you establish good sleep habits, your body and mind will be ready to perform optimally, without the strain of exhaustion. Additionally, sleeping well helps you to retain information better, so you're more likely to recall the answers when you see the test questions.

Getting good sleep means more than going to bed on time. It's important to allow your brain time to relax. Take study breaks from time to time so it doesn't get overworked, and don't study right before bed. Take time to rest your mind before trying to rest your body, or you may find it difficult to fall asleep.

Along with sleep, other aspects of physical health are important in preparing for a test. Good nutrition is vital for good brain function. Sugary foods and drinks may give a burst of energy but this burst is followed by a crash, both physically and emotionally. Instead, fuel your body with protein and vitamin-rich foods.

Also, drink plenty of water. Dehydration can lead to headaches and exhaustion, especially if your brain is already under stress from the rigors of the test. Particularly if your test is a long one, drink water during the breaks. And if possible, take an energy-boosting snack to eat between sections.

Along with sleep and diet, a third important part of physical health is exercise. Maintaining a steady workout schedule is helpful, but even taking 5-minute study breaks to walk can help get your blood pumping faster and clear your head. Exercise also releases endorphins, which contribute to a positive feeling and can help combat test anxiety.

When you nurture your physical health, you are also contributing to your mental health. If your body is healthy, your mind is much more likely to be healthy as well. So take time to rest, nourish your body with healthy food and water, and get moving as much as possible. Taking these physical steps will make you stronger and more able to take the mental steps necessary to overcome test anxiety.

Mental Steps for Beating Test Anxiety

Working on the mental side of test anxiety can be more challenging, but as with the physical side, there are clear steps you can take to overcome it. As mentioned earlier, test anxiety often stems from lack of preparation, so the obvious solution is to prepare for the test. Effective studying may be the most important weapon you have for beating test anxiety, but you can and should employ several other mental tools to combat fear.

First, boost your confidence by reminding yourself of past success—tests or projects that you aced. If you're putting as much effort into preparing for this test as you did for those, there's no reason you should expect to fail here. Work hard to prepare; then trust your preparation.

Second, surround yourself with encouraging people. It can be helpful to find a study group, but be sure that the people you're around will encourage a positive attitude. If you spend time with others who are anxious or cynical, this will only contribute to your own anxiety. Look for others who are motivated to study hard from a desire to succeed, not from a fear of failure.

Third, reward yourself. A test is physically and mentally tiring, even without anxiety, and it can be helpful to have something to look forward to. Plan an activity following the test, regardless of the outcome, such as going to a movie or getting ice cream.

When you are taking the test, if you find yourself beginning to feel anxious, remind yourself that you know the material. Visualize successfully completing the test. Then take a few deep, relaxing breaths and return to it. Work through the questions carefully but with confidence, knowing that you are capable of succeeding.

Developing a healthy mental approach to test taking will also aid in other areas of life. Test anxiety affects more than just the actual test—it can be damaging to your mental health and even contribute to depression. It's important to beat test anxiety before it becomes a problem for more than testing.

Study Strategy

Being prepared for the test is necessary to combat anxiety, but what does being prepared look like? You may study for hours on end and still not feel prepared. What you need is a strategy for test prep. The next few pages outline our recommended steps to help you plan out and conquer the challenge of preparation.

Step 1: Scope Out the Test

Learn everything you can about the format (multiple choice, essay, etc.) and what will be on the test. Gather any study materials, course outlines, or sample exams that may be available. Not only will this help you to prepare, but knowing what to expect can help to alleviate test anxiety.

Step 2: Map Out the Material

Look through the textbook or study guide and make note of how many chapters or sections it has. Then divide these over the time you have. For example, if a book has 15 chapters and you have five days to study, you need to cover three chapters each day. Even better, if you have the time, leave an extra day at the end for overall review after you have gone through the material in depth.

If time is limited, you may need to prioritize the material. Look through it and make note of which sections you think you already have a good grasp on, and which need review. While you are studying, skim quickly through the familiar sections and take more time on the challenging parts. Write out your plan so you don't get lost as you go. Having a written plan also helps you feel more in control of the study, so anxiety is less likely to arise from feeling overwhelmed at the amount to cover.

Step 3: Gather Your Tools

Decide what study method works best for you. Do you prefer to highlight in the book as you study and then go back over the highlighted portions? Or do you type out notes of the important information? Or is it helpful to make flashcards that you can carry with you? Assemble the pens, index cards, highlighters, post-it notes, and any other materials you may need so you won't be distracted by getting up to find things while you study.

If you're having a hard time retaining the information or organizing your notes, experiment with different methods. For example, try color-coding by subject with colored pens, highlighters, or post-it notes. If you learn better by hearing, try recording yourself reading your notes so you can listen while in the car, working out, or simply sitting at your desk. Ask a friend to quiz you from your flashcards, or try teaching someone the material to solidify it in your mind.

Step 4: Create Your Environment

It's important to avoid distractions while you study. This includes both the obvious distractions like visitors and the subtle distractions like an uncomfortable chair (or a too-comfortable couch that makes you want to fall asleep). Set up the best study environment possible: good lighting and a comfortable work area. If background music helps you focus, you may want to turn it on, but otherwise keep the room quiet. If you are using a computer to take notes, be sure you don't have any other windows open, especially applications like social media, games, or anything else that could distract you. Silence your phone and turn off notifications. Be sure to keep water close by so you stay hydrated while you study (but avoid unhealthy drinks and snacks).

Also, take into account the best time of day to study. Are you freshest first thing in the morning? Try to set aside some time then to work through the material. Is your mind clearer in the afternoon or evening? Schedule your study session then. Another method is to study at the same time of day that you will take the test, so that your brain gets used to working on the material at that time and will be ready to focus at test time.

Step 5: Study!

Once you have done all the study preparation, it's time to settle into the actual studying. Sit down, take a few moments to settle your mind so you can focus, and begin to follow your study plan. Don't give in to distractions or let yourself procrastinate. This is your time to prepare so you'll be ready to fearlessly approach the test. Make the most of the time and stay focused.

Of course, you don't want to burn out. If you study too long you may find that you're not retaining the information very well. Take regular study breaks. For example, taking five minutes out of every hour to walk briskly, breathing deeply and swinging your arms, can help your mind stay fresh.

As you get to the end of each chapter or section, it's a good idea to do a quick review. Remind yourself of what you learned and work on any difficult parts. When you feel that you've mastered the material, move on to the next part. At the end of your study session, briefly skim through your notes again.

But while review is helpful, cramming last minute is NOT. If at all possible, work ahead so that you won't need to fit all your study into the last day. Cramming overloads your brain with more information than it can process and retain, and your tired mind may struggle to recall even previously learned information when it is overwhelmed with last-minute study. Also, the urgent nature of cramming and the stress placed on your brain contribute to anxiety. You'll be more likely to go to the test feeling unprepared and having trouble thinking clearly.

So don't cram, and don't stay up late before the test, even just to review your notes at a leisurely pace. Your brain needs rest more than it needs to go over the information again. In fact, plan to finish your studies by noon or early afternoon the day before the test. Give your brain the rest of the day to relax or focus on other things, and get a good night's sleep. Then you will be fresh for the test and better able to recall what you've studied.

Step 6: Take a Practice Test

Many courses offer sample tests, either online or in the study materials. This is an excellent resource to check whether you have mastered the material, as well as to prepare for the test format and environment.

Check the test format ahead of time: the number of questions, the type (multiple choice, free response, etc.), and the time limit. Then create a plan for working through them. For example, if you have 30 minutes to take a 60-question test, your limit is 30 seconds per question. Spend less time on the questions you know well so that you can take more time on the difficult ones.

If you have time to take several practice tests, take the first one open book, with no time limit. Work through the questions at your own pace and make sure you fully understand them. Gradually work up to taking a test under test conditions: sit at a desk with all study materials put away and set a timer. Pace yourself to make sure you finish the test with time to spare and go back to check your answers if you have time.

After each test, check your answers. On the questions you missed, be sure you understand why you missed them. Did you misread the question (tests can use tricky wording)? Did you forget the information? Or was it something you hadn't learned? Go back and study any shaky areas that the practice tests reveal.

Taking these tests not only helps with your grade, but also aids in combating test anxiety. If you're already used to the test conditions, you're less likely to worry about it, and working through tests until you're scoring well gives you a confidence boost. Go through the practice tests until you feel comfortable, and then you can go into the test knowing that you're ready for it.

Test Tips

On test day, you should be confident, knowing that you've prepared well and are ready to answer the questions. But aside from preparation, there are several test day strategies you can employ to maximize your performance.

First, as stated before, get a good night's sleep the night before the test (and for several nights before that, if possible). Go into the test with a fresh, alert mind rather than staying up late to study.

Try not to change too much about your normal routine on the day of the test. It's important to eat a nutritious breakfast, but if you normally don't eat breakfast at all, consider eating just a protein bar. If you're a coffee drinker, go ahead and have your normal coffee. Just make sure you time it so that the caffeine doesn't wear off right in the middle of your test. Avoid sugary beverages, and drink enough water to stay hydrated but not so much that you need a restroom break 10 minutes into the test. If your test isn't first thing in the morning, consider going for a walk or doing a light workout before the test to get your blood flowing.

Allow yourself enough time to get ready, and leave for the test with plenty of time to spare so you won't have the anxiety of scrambling to arrive in time. Another reason to be early is to select a good seat. It's helpful to sit away from doors and windows, which can be distracting. Find a good seat, get out your supplies, and settle your mind before the test begins.

When the test begins, start by going over the instructions carefully, even if you already know what to expect. Make sure you avoid any careless mistakes by following the directions.

Then begin working through the questions, pacing yourself as you've practiced. If you're not sure on an answer, don't spend too much time on it, and don't let it shake your confidence. Either skip it and come back later, or eliminate as many wrong answers as possible and guess among the remaining ones. Don't dwell on these questions as you continue—put them out of your mind and focus on what lies ahead.

Be sure to read all of the answer choices, even if you're sure the first one is the right answer. Sometimes you'll find a better one if you keep reading. But don't second-guess yourself if you do immediately know the answer. Your gut instinct is usually right. Don't let test anxiety rob you of the information you know.

If you have time at the end of the test (and if the test format allows), go back and review your answers. Be cautious about changing any, since your first instinct tends to be correct, but make sure you didn't misread any of the questions or accidentally mark the wrong answer choice. Look over any you skipped and make an educated guess.

At the end, leave the test feeling confident. You've done your best, so don't waste time worrying about your performance or wishing you could change anything. Instead, celebrate the successful completion of this test. And finally, use this test to learn how to deal with anxiety even better next time.

Review Video: Test Anxiety
Visit mometrix.com/academy and enter code: 100340

Important Qualification

Not all anxiety is created equal. If your test anxiety is causing major issues in your life beyond the classroom or testing center, or if you are experiencing troubling physical symptoms related to your anxiety, it may be a sign of a serious physiological or psychological condition. If this sounds like your situation, we strongly encourage you to seek professional help.

Online Resources

Due to our efforts to try to keep this book to a manageable length, we've created a link that will give you access to all of your online resources:

mometrix.com/resources719/ardmsobgyn

It's Your Moment, Let's Celebrate It!

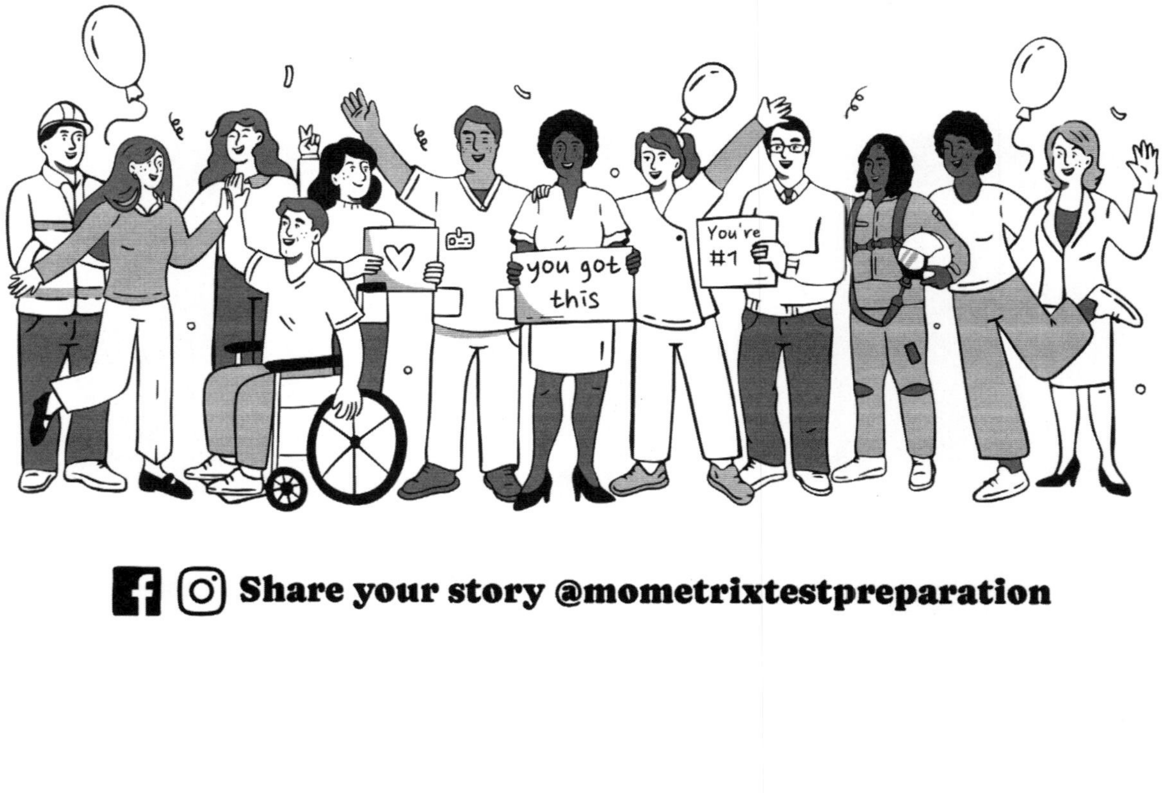

Share your story @mometrixtestpreparation